Food and Drink in Archaeology 3
University of Nottingham Postgraduate Conference 2009

Food and Drink in Archaeology 3

University of Nottingham Postgraduate Conference 2009

Edited by
Dave Collard, Jim Morris and Elisa Perego

Prospect Books
2012

First published in Great Britain in 2012 by Prospect Books, Allaleigh House, Blackawton, Totnes, Devon, TQ9 7DL.

© 2012 as a collection Prospect Books.
© 2012 in individual articles rests with the authors.

The authors assert their moral right to be identified as authors in accordance with the Copyright, Designs & Patents Act 1988. No part of this publication may be reproduced, stored in a retrieval system or transmitted in any form or by any means, electronic, mechanical, photocopying, recording or otherwise, without the prior permission of the copyright holders.

ISBN 978-1-903018-78-1

The illustration on the cover is courtesy of the University of Nottingham Archaeology Museum.

For more information about Prospect Books: https://www.prospectbooks.co.uk.

Design and typesetting in Gill Sans and Adobe Garamond by Tom Jaine & O. Pawley.
Printed and bound in Great Britain by Jellyfish Solutions, Southampton.

Contents

List of Figures — 7

Preface — 11

Cemetery, Ceramics and Space: Food Consumption and Ritual at the Early Bronze Age Tholos Cemetery of Moni Odigitria, South Central Greece
Tim Campbell-Green and Flora Michelaki — 13

Drinking with the Dead: Pyschoactive Consumption in Cypriote Bronze Age Mortuary Ritual
Dave Collard — 23

Symbols of the Feasts: Élite Ideology and Feasting Practices in Early Iron Age Greece
Rachel Fox — 33

Intoxicating Drinks and Drunkards in Ancient Indian Art, Literature and Archaeology
Nitin Hadap and Shilpa Hadap — 41

A New Renaissance Medical Controversy: Sixteenth-Century Polemics About Cold-Drinking
Justo Hernández — 47

Living and Eating in Coastal Brazil During Prehistory
Mercedes Okumura and Sabine Eggers — 55

Between Sacrifice and Consumption: the Deceased as Metaphorical Food in Iron Age Veneto
Elisa Perego — 65

A Different Kettle of Fish: Food Diversity in Mesolithic Scotland
Catriona Pickard and Clive Bonsall — 76

The Recognition and Interpretation of a Singular Late Bronze Age Animal Sacrifice Event at Kilise Tepe, Turkey
Peter Popkin — 89

Triple Cups and Bird-Shaped Pottery: Ritualized Feasting-Goods from Norwegian Graves Dating from the First to the Fifth Centuries AD
Christian Rødsrud 99

Animals in the Household: Not Just a Foodstuff
Aixa Vidal and Ruth Maicas 111

Feasting and the State in Uruk Mesopotamia
Jessica Whalen 119

Shorter Contributions

Cleaning Grain and Making Beer: Analysis of a Third- to Fourth-Century AD Archaeobotanical Assemblage from Bottisham, Cambridge
Kate Parks 127

The Fauna of the Neolithic Lakeside Settlement of Dispilio, Greek Macedonia
Eleni Samartzidou 133

Eating, Processing and Storing Food in Arid Andean Highlands
Aixa Vidal 139

Prehistoric Spoons: Their Representation in Time and Space
Aixa Vidal and M. Soledad Mallía 144

List of Figures

1.1	Approximate dates for the Cretan Early and Middle Bronze Age periods, based on Manning (1995)	14
1.2	Plan of the Early Bronze Age Cemetery of Moni Odigitria, Southern Crete (courtesy of Dr Antonis Vasilakis, additional captions by the authors)	15
1.3	Early Bronze IIB shallow open bowls or plates (drawings by the authors)	17
1.4	Early Bronze Cooking Pot Ware one-handled cups/scoops (drawings by the authors)	17
2.1	Base Ring juglets from Kazaphani-Ayios Andronikos Tomb 2 (after Nikolaou & Nikolaou 1989, Pl. XI)	25
2.2	Opium poppy head compared with a Base Ring I juglet (after Merrillees 1962, Pl. XLII)	26
2.3	Hawkes' 'Ladder of Inference' (D. Collard)	27
5.1	Title page of *Pedacio Dioscórides...* edited and translated by Andrés Laguna (Biblioteca Histórica 'Marqués de Valdecilla', Madrid)	49
5.2	Title page of *Tractado de la nieve...* by Francisco Franco (Biblioteca Histórica 'Marqués de Valdecilla', Madrid)	51
5.3	Title page of *Libro que trata de la nieve...* by Nicolás Monardes (Biblioteca Histórica 'Marqués de Valdecilla', Madrid)	52
6.1	a) map of Brazil presenting the area shown in greater detail in d; b) polished stone figurine representing fish; c) shellmound site; d) detail of map showing states (RJ: Rio de Janeiro; SP: Sao Paulo; PR: Parana; SC: Santa Catarina) and location of sites mentioned in the article (1: Beirada; 2: Tenorio; 3: Piacaguera; 4: Forte Marechal Luz, Enseada I, Itacoara, Ilha de Espinheiros II, Morro do Ouro, and Rio Comprido; 5: Cabecuda and Jabuticabeira II)	56
6.2	Percentage of teeth affected by caries per site (after Okumura and Eggers 2005, 269; Scheel-Ybert et al. 2003, 120). 'Rio Comprido Upper' and 'Rio Comprido Lower' refer to skeletons found in upper and lower layers of the same site	60
6.3	Percentage of osteoarthritis (OA) observed in arms and legs in different	

	sites (after Okumura and Eggers 2005, 270; Petronilho 2003, 88). 'Rio Comprido Upper' and 'Rio Comprido Lower' refer to skeletons found in upper and lower layers of the same site	61
7.1	Map of Veneto with sites mentioned in the chapter (drawn by the author)	67
7.2	Grave assemblage from infant Gazzo Vr. Colombara tomb 34 (900–850 BC): biconical vessel used as urn; large bowl used as a lid; small bowl; arched fibula; ring and pierced shell valve (modified by the author after Salzani 2001)	67
7.3	Total number of urns attested per class of vessels (drawn by the author)	69
8.1	Sites mentioned in the text	77
8.2	Radiocarbon determinations of sites mentioned in text (from Ashmore 2004)	78
8.3	Oronsay human bone collagen stable isotope values (from Richards and Mellars 1998, table 1)	81
9.1	Sheep skeleton deposited in pit P08/23 (photograph by the author)	91
9.2	Heavily butchered axis vertebrae dorsal (left) and right side (right) views (photographs courtesy Bob Miller)	92
10.1	Triple cups of pottery (a–c) and wood (d–e), all drawings are out of scale: a) Mus. no. C21408, Hedrum prestegård, Larvik, Vestfold, Norway, AD 350–450 (drawing by Skafft); b) Mus. no. C30491g, Trålum, Fjære, Aust-Agder, Norway, AD 350–450 (drawing by unknown); c) Mus. no. C29860b, Ula, Fredrikstad, Østfold, Norway, probably AD 100–300 (drawing by Tone Strenger); d) Telemark, Norway, eighteenth century (after Gjærder 1975, fig. 242); e) Telemark, Norway, seventeenth/eighteenth century (photograph by the author)	100
10.2	Bird-shaped beakers: a) Mus. no. S1413–1422, Bjerkreim, Helleland, Rogaland, Norway, AD 350–450 (photograph, Museum of Archaeology, University of Stavanger); b) Mus. no. C29264, Ås østre, Sande, Vestfold, Norway, AD 300–400 (photograph by the author); c) the docks, Bergen, Norway, fourteenth century (after Gjærder 1975, fig. 255); d) Nissedal, Telemark, Norway, eighteenth century (after Gjærder 1975, fig. 256)	104
10.3	Set of three vessels from Ås østre, Sande, Vestfold, Norway, AD 300–400 (photograph by the author)	106
11.1	Some tools made of animal materials from Almizaraque (Almería):	

	a) pointed tools; b) arrowpoint; c) button; d) shell vessel with ochre; e) oculated idol on rib bone	113
11.2	Siret's drawing of the Cista de Mina Ibéria (Almería). Argaric burial with an important offering of meat (bovid tibia)	114
11.3	Bone structure recorded in Siret's notebooks	115
12.1	Map showing sites mentioned in the text	120
12.2	Perforated plaque from Nippur featuring droop-spouted jar (after Boese 1971, Plate 18, 8)	122
13.1	The larger 'corndrier' (photograph by Archaeological Solutions)	128
13.2	i) Weed autecological indication of soil nitrogen content; ii) weed perennation; iii) weed autecological indication of soil acidity	129
13.3	Crop processing sequence (numbers indicate number of samples representing each stage)	130
14.1	Map of western and central Macedonia showing the site of Dispilio	133
14.2	Composition of the identified assemblage from Dispilio in terms of NISP (Number of Identified Specimens)	135
14.3	Ageing data for Dispilio sheep/goats shown against Payne's (1973) 'meat' model	137
15.1	Location of Casa Chávez Montículos in Antofagasta de la Sierra (Catamarca, Argentina)	140
15.2	Representation of the different ceramic groups in Casa Chávez Montículos during its two phases	141
16.1	Different terms used in the literature for spoon-shaped artefacts and their associated residues	145
16.2	The temporal distribution of spoons and their materials of manufacture	146
16.3	The main records of spoons in prehistoric Europe and neighbouring areas, highlighted according to raw material (Vidal and Mallía forthcoming)	147

Preface

The third Food and Drink in Archaeology conference took place at the University of Nottingham 17–18 April 2009 and, as ever, was attended by scholars from a wide geographical range and with equally diverse research interests. Over the course of the two days, 24 papers were delivered across five sessions: the first on the identification of feasting and consumption events, the second on the link between food and the dead, the third on the archaeology of drinking, the fourth on culture change, with a general session sponsored by the Association for Environmental Archaeology.

This volume reproduces half of the papers that were delivered at the conference, together with four shorter articles that have been developed from posters. The contents are exceptionally international, with chapters examining evidence from northern and southern Europe, the Near East, India and the Americas, and research spans the mesolithic to post-medieval periods. Whilst the content is largely archaeological, many of the chapters are interdisciplinary in their approach, drawing on evidence from (art) history as well as anthropology and the hard sciences.

All of the papers were subject to peer review and we are grateful to the many scholars who took the time to provide such full assessments and detailed advice, both to the authors and to us as editors. We should also like to thank the University of Nottingham's Annual Fund, who provided financial support to enable the publication of the proceedings. Once again, thanks are due to our publisher, Tom Jaine of Prospect Books, for his help and patience.

Dave Collard, *University of Nottingham*

Jim Morris, *Museum of London Archaeological Service*

Elisa Perego, *University College, London*

Cemetery, Ceramics and Space: Food Consumption and Ritual at the Early Bronze Age Tholos Cemetery of Moni Odigitria, South Central Crete

*Tim Campbell-Green, University of Sheffield
and Flora Michelaki, University College, London*

In recent years it has been proposed that food consumption and feasting practices, beyond those associated with the day-to-day calorific intake, were important – possibly central – facets of life in the Aegean Bronze Age and, in particular, on the island of Crete (e.g. Hamilakis 1998; 2000; Day and Wilson 2004). Crete has an extremely rich and complex archaeological heritage that has allowed commensal food consumption to be explored in a number of different contexts and with regard to a variety of purposes and functions, notably within the palaces and wider palatial society of the Middle and Late Bronze Age (Day and Wilson 1998; 2002). For the earlier periods, evidence for feasting practices has been less forthcoming, although it has been suggested that commensal consumption took place within Early Bronze Age tholos tombs (Hamilakis 1998).

Confined largely, but not exclusively, to the south-central area of the island, the tholos tombs of Early Bronze Age Crete are particular forms of large vaulted structures used for multiple communal burials. They are characterized by a circular plan, a (commonly) east-facing doorway, antechambers built onto the external wall of the tomb, and frequently an external courtyard area. They begin to be built in the EB I period and continue until the earlier part of the Middle Bronze Age, with sporadic use noted after that. Indeed, their longevity is such that some individual tombs were in constant use for burials for over 1000 years – an astonishing endurance of use and tradition (see Branigan 1993 for a general overview of the tholos tombs). The material culture associated with these cemeteries is typified by large quantities of pottery, as well as other items such as gold and stone jewellery, stone vessels and metalwork. Occasionally, material that may be classed as 'ritual paraphernalia' – e.g. libation vessels, anthropo- or zoomorphic vessels and statues – are recovered, in addition to objects that may be said to be associated with everyday life such as razors, knives, or beads. Most commonly encountered are ceramic vessels of all types and forms, and whilst some were probably just grave-goods, in the traditional sense of accompanying the deceased in the tomb, the majority were seemingly employed in the consumption of food and drink.

The idea of consumption at the tombs was first noted in 1924 (Xanthoudides 1924); however, it was with the publication of *Tombs of the Mesara* (Branigan 1970) that a more active role for the pottery in a tholos cemetery was proposed. As a significant number of cups are found at all tombs, often in small and discrete groups, a form of toasting ritual was hypothesized as a post-interment rite, involving a select number of people and small cups of, presumably, wine. Thus, whilst the consumption of drink has been acknowledged as a feature of ritual activity at the tombs, there has been very little evidence for role of consumption within the cemetery beyond this. However, this paper will discuss recent work on the Cretan cemetery of Moni Odigitria, which has shown that consumption, above and beyond the toasting rite, was indeed occurring, and that it may have formed a central practice in the ritual life of the cemetery (Branigan and Campbell-Green 2010; Campbell-Green 2006).

In terms of chronology, the Cretan Neolithic and Bronze Age is notoriously complex but a rough outline of absolute dates for the Cretan Early and Middle Bronze Age periods, based on Manning (1995), is provided below.

Cultural Group	*Approximate Date*
Early Minoan I	3100–2700 BC
Early Minoan IIA	2700–2450 BC
Early Minoan IIB	2450–2200 BC
Early Minoan III	2200–2100 BC
Middle Minoan IA	2100–1900 BC
Middle Minoan IB	1900–1800 BC
Middle Minoan IIA	1800–1750 BC
Middle Minoan IIB	1750–1700 BC

Figure 1.1. Approximate dates for the Cretan Early and Middle Bronze Age periods, based on Manning (1995).

The Tholos Cemetery at Moni Odigitria

Located on the lower slopes of the Asterousia mountains in south-central Crete, Moni Odigitria is a typical example of the tholos cemetery type (Figure 1.2).

It comprises two tombs, A and B, enclosed by a peribolos 'wall' which marks the extent of the cemetery. It was used, probably continuously, for a period of not less than 800 years – beginning life in the EB I period with the construction of Tomb A. Measuring 3.5m in diameter, Tomb A was a relatively simple, free-standing structure that remained in use until it was seemingly abandoned in EB II for reasons that are unclear. The larger Tomb B was built at this point, probably to replace the function of Tomb A, and demonstrates a greater complexity in its structure, more typical of the tomb type. Measuring some 6m in diameter, it is surrounded by open 'courtyards' laid out within the peribolos, and has a suite of three anterooms situated in front of the entrance,

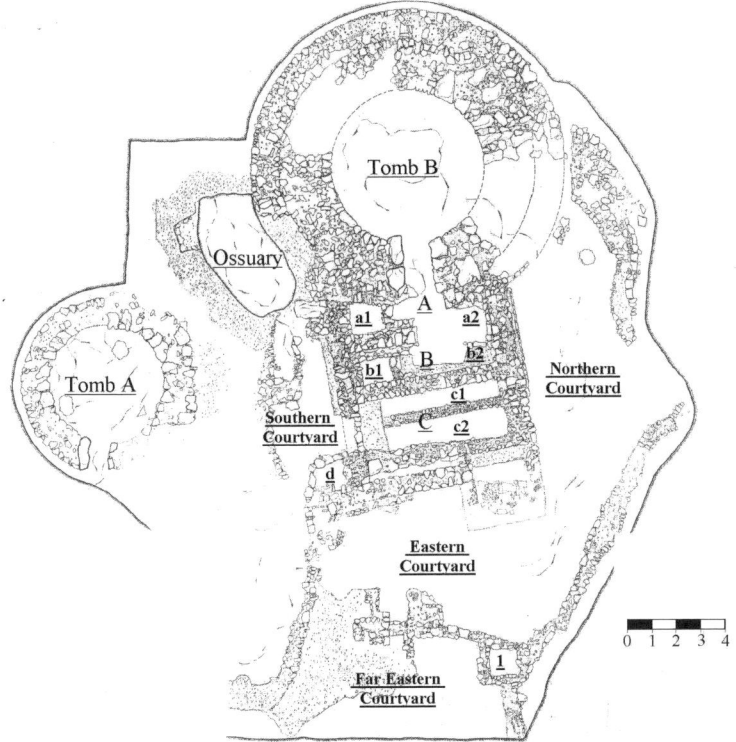

Figure 1.2. Plan of the Early Bronze Age Cemetery of Moni Odigitria, southern Crete (courtesy of Dr Antonis Vasilakis, additional captions by the authors).

through which access to the tomb-proper was gained. Construction and reconstruction continued at Tomb B until it was finally abandoned in the MB I period.

The cemetery was, regrettably, looted prior to excavation in 1979/1980; the interior of both tombs had been removed – completely in the case of Tomb B, with only a small strip remaining in the case of Tomb A. Although the looters had dug several relatively small-scale pits outside the tomb chambers, it seems there was little other disturbance of the archaeological levels within the *ca.* 340m² of open space between and around the tombs. As a result, a substantial proportion of the vessels were still in the place they were used and deposited in the Bronze Age. Careful excavation of the cemetery coupled with the retention and study of the complete ceramic assemblage recovered, has yielded a significant body of data with which to work. The cemetery produced a total of some 66,000 pottery sherds, weighing just less than one metric ton and representing a minimum of 6000 vessels ranging in date from EB I to MB II. This assemblage is one of the largest excavated from a tholos cemetery, and perhaps as much as a third of it has a secure archaeological context. Importantly, the excellent condition of preservation and excavation within the cemetery has allowed a diachronic and spatial analysis of the assemblage that has revealed a number of interesting and significant patterns, to which we now turn (Michelaki and Campbell-Green forthcoming).

The Ceramic Evidence

Perhaps the most obvious trend apparent in the ceramic assemblage is the consistent and increasing emphasis on drinking vessels. This, clearly, suggests that the consumption of drink was a central aspect of ritual practice during the life of the cemetery. The nature of the drink-related rites in the early periods is unclear but, judging from the pottery recovered from within this and other tombs, it may be that they were concentrated on the interior of the tomb itself. By the MB I, however, it is apparent that a toasting ritual was also being performed in the anterooms.

A second interesting trend in the ceramic evidence relates to the representation of food-associated vessels: their relative frequency increases dramatically from less than five per cent in the EB I and MB I, to around 20 per cent in the EB IIB. This substantial rise in food-related vessels is in large part due to the emergence of new vessels such as the shallow open bowl/plate types (Fig. 1.3).

The meaning of this shift in ceramic representation is uncertain but it probably reflects a change in the way rites were performed at the cemetery; perhaps an elaboration of the earlier basic toasting practices. It might also be connected with the emergence of the 'individual' as a participant in the rituals at this time, and the corresponding change in material culture that accompanied it. For instance, where in the EB I and early EB II chalices and pedestalled bowls had probably served as communal vessels (an interpretation suggested by their large size), the later vessels show a marked reduction in volume that rendered them usable only for individual service (Day and Wilson 2004).

Associated with this EB II increase in food vessels is the large quantity of Cooking Pot Ware, which was recovered from all areas of the cemetery and constitutes 10 per cent of the ceramic assemblage. Cooking Pot Ware is one of the more commonly encountered ware types in Bronze Age settlements (Vasilakis forthcoming) and appears to have been central to domestic life. It is not, however, normally found in any great quantity from cemetery contexts. For instance, at Ayia Kyriaki (Blackman and Branigan 1982), a similarly dated cemetery in the next valley along, only a few Cooking Pot Ware sherds were present, comprising just 0.3 per cent of the assemblage. Clearly then, at Moni Odigitria something different was occurring. Much of the Cooking Pot Ware was fragmentary, but a number of forms are present: the shallow baking platter (of which only rims were recovered), large pedestalled bowls, open bowls, rare examples of tripod cooking pots and, the most commonly encountered, the one-handled cup or scoop (Fig. 1.4).

Cooking Pot Ware is somewhat difficult to date because the forms are conservative, so cannot generally be dated on stylistic grounds alone, and the nature of the contexts proscribes simple dating by deposit. However, associated pottery deposits, as well as parallels from elsewhere on the island, suggest that much of Moni Odigitria's material

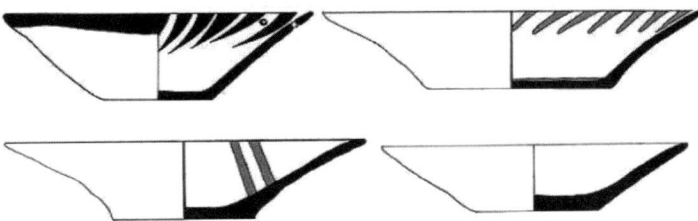

Figure 1.3. Early Bronze IIB shallow open bowls or plates (drawings by the authors).

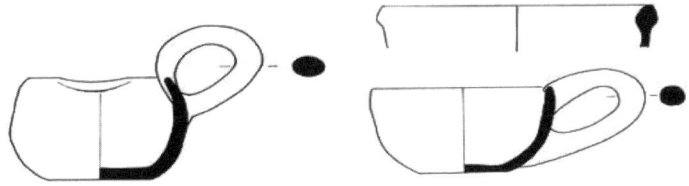

Figure 1.4. Early Bronze Cooking Pot Ware one-handled cups/scoops (drawings by the authors).

is EB II in date. Importantly, whilst Cooking Pot Ware can be used for a number of things (e.g. storage or as lamps), as much as 40 per cent of that recovered showed clear, localized, burn marks, and had obviously been used for cooking prior to deposition within the cemetery (Campbell-Green forthcoming).

Although found in consistently small quantities throughout the cemetery, one specific area was particularly rich in Cooking Pot Ware: the far eastern courtyard. It is this area that may allow us to understand not only the meaning of this pottery type but also how the cemetery was used. From this courtyard area, paved with compacted stone, Cooking Pot Ware accounted for more than 16 per cent of all vessels, nearly double the average for the cemetery. In the centre of the courtyard was a large and spatially distinct patch of burnt earth and charcoal, measuring one metre square and 0.15m deep – the so-called 'Burnt Deposit'. This was kept as a separate context by the excavator and analysis revealed that Cooking Pot Ware accounted for 24 per cent of vessels from this deposit.

Taken together, the evidence (i.e. the frequency of cooking vessels, the fact that many showed characteristic burn marks and their association with the 'Burnt Deposit') strongly indicates that cooking occurred within the courtyard of the cemetery complex. Other smaller patches of burnt earth and charcoal were noted in the courtyard, and it is likely that these too were cooking fires; however, the size and depth of the Burnt Deposit, together with the large number of vessels it contained, suggests this hearth was favoured and used repeatedly for episodes of food preparation. It seems, then, that this area acted as the location for the preparation and serving of food and drink, with consumption taking place elsewhere in the cemetery, probably in the courtyards surrounding the tomb. The use of this preparation area appears to have lasted until the EB II, as by the MB I the far eastern courtyard had been largely abandoned and food-associated vessels virtually disappear. In their place there is a re-emergence of drinking vessels and activity shifts to the anterooms, suggesting a return to drinking rites within the cemetery.

What, then, is the meaning of such activity, and how are we to interpret both the consumption of food, and the presence of the pottery littering the cemetery in such quantities?

An important concept that allows us to better understand the tombs is that of the cemetery as a 'heterotopia' – a liminal place simultaneously part of, but clearly removed from, the normal, everyday world.

The Cemetery as a Heterotopia

That the tombs were located near to their contributing settlement (Vasilakis forthcoming), and not placed far away or out of view, illustrates that the cemeteries were not considered unknown or 'distant' places without any connection to domestic life in the physical sense. And yet, the presence of the tombs themselves – the formalized structure as distinct places of interment, the use of an above-ground structure and its permanency, the 'plugging in' of this place into the wider environment, the presence of many generations of the dead, and through this the relationship of the dead to the living – imply extra-normal activity. Therefore, and conversely, the cemeteries were simultaneously understood as being different from the settlements and, given their primary use, conceptualized as 'special' places set apart from everyday life and imbued with a heterotopic quality; they became what Thomas (1993, 77–8) terms a 'dominant locale'. This quality may have been augmented by conceptual definition and construction – the area is set apart through taboo, avoidance, and a tacit understanding of its meaning and importance – concepts that are noted in a number of ethnographic studies of death and burial (e.g. Bloch 1971).

Such differentiation was also emphasized by more tangible, physical, separation. For instance, the shape and size of the tomb would not only have drawn attention to the existence of the cemetery from a distance but would also have set it apart from the surrounding landscape. Separation would have been enhanced further by deliberate modifications – such as paving, flattening or the use of different coloured earth – to the area around the tomb, or, as at Moni Odigitria and elsewhere, through the erection of a wall. In cases where there is no obvious evidence for modification, it seems possible that archaeologically invisible methods – reeds, animal skins or other type of organic fencing – may have been employed.

This ambiguity in conceptual location and difficulty in categorization associated with the tombs, coupled with its obvious association with the dead, may have resulted in the cemetery taking on the status as a place where the living could connect or interact, physically or symbolically, with the dead and/or the supernatural. Moreover, repeated ritual and burial action within the cemetery must have led the tombs to develop a 'history', becoming a place sanctified through tradition. In this manner, through their identification as being conceptually 'different', the cemeteries would have functioned as a means of 'locating the subject in relation to both the physical and metaphysical world' (Thomas 1993, 81).

It is this concept, then, of the cemetery as a heterotopia, that allows us to explore further the role of the cemeteries within the cosmology of the tomb builders and users, and their relationships to, and perceptions of, the dead. The action of eating takes on new meaning and resonance within this heterotopic context. Whilst eating is a normal activity, it is not normal to eat in a cemetery, and to do so emphasizes difference and the specialness of both place and activity. The action of eating in this instance may be associated with mnemonics and concepts of remembering/forgetting such as those suggested by Hamilakis (1998). Thus, we should perhaps begin to think more about the types of food and drink being consumed: are they 'normal', everyday foodstuffs, or are they 'special' in terms of meaning or ingredients, perhaps containing psychoactive properties to facilitate communication with the divine or the dead (see Collard, this volume).

The use of vessels in this heterotopic space may explain why they were left *in situ* – tainted and transformed through function and location – so that they could not be reused in a profane manner at a later date (Webb 1992, 88). As a result the ground became strewn with pottery, both whole vessels and sherds, which altered the shape, texture and colour of the area – emphasizing further its heterotopic quality. Moreover, the pottery acts as a means of 'presencing' the past activity, and thus the past meanings, into the present, and becomes a metaphor for the dead – a way of representing the individual through a material symbol (Thomas 1993, 77). Indeed, on a metaphysical level, we may suggest that the consumption of food and drink fixes a particular event within a temporal and spatial framework that enables that particular event to be recalled at a later date. Simultaneously, however, previous events are in turn recalled in this manner, and so the cycle of remembrance continues, manipulating both time and space through the use and presence of pottery.

It could be, thus, suggested that activity at the tombs repeated over many generations serves to reinforce the link between the living and the dead, the past and the present – a link made all the more powerful if the remains of these past activities lie literally at their feet.

As a means of illustrating the conceptual complexity and powerful meaning that may have driven and informed funerary activity in the Early Bronze Age, as well as placing this activity into a cultural context, we would like to suggest a similarity in action, purpose and meaning between the cemeteries in the Bronze Age, with funerary and post-funerary activity in contemporary Cretan society. By this, we do not wish to infer that there is an unbroken chain in tradition and custom from the Minoan period to the present: that would be unrealistic, unlikely and unimprovable. Rather, that such activity reflects a human need evident in all societies and in all periods.

Funerary Rituals in Contemporary Crete

The most obvious, and most commonly observed, rituals associated with the dead in contemporary Crete are those of the 'remembrance days' – post-funerary memorial services that occur at set intervals following the death of an individual. The first remembrance service takes place three days after death (this is considered the most significant for the deceased), with others following at nine days, forty days, three months, six months, nine months and one year; each one is considered important and observed with the utmost solemnity. The ceremonies normally take place in the morning at a church near the cemetery, after which people gather in an area next to the cemetery to consume food and drink in memory of the dead. Although this has become the most common method of observing these rites, in a small number of villages in the south of the island it is still the tradition for these memorials to take place within the cemetery, especially in the Mesara and Malevizi regions. Here, food and drink is brought to the cemetery, and even prepared among the graves, and people gather at the graveside to eat and drink on top of the grave itself. Indeed, in order to facilitate these food consumption events, equipment, utensils and condiments are sometimes stored at the cemeteries. Such occasions are known as *Nekrodeipna*, or 'dead meals', and by tradition occur on the first Saturday of Lent. The custom is most common in the Mesara region and in the Malevizi area, although *Nekrodeipna* are becoming increasingly rare even in these villages. The custom of bringing food to the tombs after Easter Sunday is more common. This tradition is explicitly linked to the Orthodox Church, and in particular it represents a connection between the resurrection of Christ on the Sunday and the rebirth of the soul of the departed in Paradise. The meal is usually made up of traditional Easter foodstuffs such as sweet cakes, bread and hard-boiled eggs that have been dyed red (Psilakis 2005, 196–197).

In general, choices about which food and drinks are consumed reflect the personal tastes of the deceased or of those taking part, but an important element of the memorial meal, eaten by all those attending, is the *kollyva* – a type of boiled wheat. The wheat symbolizes the 'resurrection' of the dead and the eternal soul in the afterlife, the idea being that, like the cycle of the seed, the dead are buried in the earth, they change form and seemingly decompose, but the essential element grows again back into life (according to Christian Orthodox tradition). The consumption of the *kollyva* is, then, a central aspect of the proceedings, serving to reassure the participants of the concept of eternal life, and to reiterate the central tenet of the magico-religious structure informing the ritual.

Finally, it has not been long since the living used to pour wine in front of the tomb. It was a form of ritual for the 'thirsty' dead. This could be seen in Petrokefali in the

Mesara region, as well as in the villages near Kissamos at Chania, where they used to bring a glass of wine during the memorial services, turn it upside down and pour the wine on the soil for forgiveness and rest for the dead (Psilakis 2005, 196). The last 30–40 years have seen these rituals and customs begin to fade.

Conclusion

Overall then, the philosophy behind the post-funerary activity in contemporary Crete is about the remembrance of the dead, and the rebirth and eternal life of the deceased, both symbolic and actual. It is through location that we see this made manifest, and through this, a form of communication between the living and the dead may be achieved. It is precisely this, we suggest, that can be observed in the Bronze Age, with the cemetery acting as a heterotopic nodal point through which communication between the worlds is enabled and within which the consumption of food and drink is a central aspect of ritual.

Considering the archaeological evidence, whatever the interpretation of the chrono–logical and spatial patterning of pottery deposition in the case of the Prepalatial cemetery at Moni Odigitria, one conclusion may be confidently drawn from our examination of this vast assemblage. Pottery was not just used and deposited as passive grave-goods alongside burials in the two tomb chambers – though doubtless this happened. Rather, pottery played an active, functional, role in many aspects of life and death and all their attendant ceremonies and rites, throughout the life of the tomb.

As for contemporary Cretan society, the repeated post-funerary rituals are the most common custom that has survived through time and gives a special significance to the memory of the dead as well as an opportunity for living relatives to pay tribute and to show their respect.

References

Blackman, D. and Branigan, K. 1982. 'The excavation of an Early Minoan Tholos tomb at Ayia Kyriaki, Ayiofarango', *Annual of the British School at Athens* 77, 1–57.

Bloch, M. 1971. *Placing The Dead* (London and New York).

Branigan, K. 1970. *The Tombs of Mesara. A Study of Funerary Architecture and Ritual in Southern Crete* (London).

—— 1993. *Dancing With Death: Life and Death in Southern Crete c. 3000 – 2000 BC* (Amsterdam).

—— and Campbell-Green, T. 2010. 'The Pottery', in Vasilakis, A. and Branigan, K. (eds) *Moni Odigitria: A Prepalatial Cemetery and its Environs in the Asterousia, Southern Crete* (Philadelphia), 69–143.

Campbell-Green, T. 2006. *Cemetery, Ceramics and Space: An Analysis of the Pottery Assemblage from the Early Minoan Cemetery of Moni Odigitria*. Unpublished PhD Thesis, Department of Prehistory and Archaeology, University of Sheffield.

—— forthcoming. 'Burnt offerings? Burn marks on vessels from the early Minoan cemetery of Moni Odigitria', in *Proceedings of the 10th International Cretological Congress* (Khania).

Day, P.M. and Wilson, D.E. 1998. 'Consuming power: Kamares Ware in Protopalatial Knossos', *Antiquity* 72, 350–358.

—— 2002. 'Landscapes of memory, craft and power in Prepalatial and Protopalatial Knossos', in Hamilakis, Y. (ed.), *Labyrinth Revisited: Rethinking 'Minoan' Archaeology* (Oxford), 143–166.

—— 2004. 'Ceramic change and the practice of eating and drinking in EBA Crete', in Halstead, P. and Barrett, J. (eds), *Food, Cuisine and Society in Prehistoric Greece* (Oxford), 45–62.

Hamilakis, Y. 1998. 'Eating the dead: mortuary feasting and the politics of memory in Aegean Bronze Age society', in Branigan, K. (ed.) *Cemetery and Society in the Aegean Bronze Age* (Sheffield), 115–132.

—— 2000. 'The anthropology of food and drink consumption and Aegean archaeology', in Vaughan, S. and Coulson, W. (eds) *Palaeodiet in the Aegean* (Oxford), 55–63.

Manning, S.W. 1995. *The Absolute Chronology of the Aegean Early Bronze Age: Archaeology, Radiocarbon and History* (Sheffield).

Michelaki, F. and Campbell-Green, T. forthcoming. 'Pottery usage at the Prepalatial cemetery of Moni Odigitria', in *Proceedings of the 10th International Cretological Congress* (Khania).

Psilakis, N. 2005. *Laikes Teletourgies Sten Kriti* (Crete).

Thomas, J. 1993. 'The hermeneutics of Megalithic space', in Tilley, C. (ed.) *Interpretative Archaeology* (Oxford), 73–97.

Vasilakis, A. forthcoming. *The Early Minoan Settlement of Trypiti*.

Webb, J.M. 1992. 'Funerary ideology in Bronze Age Cyprus – toward the recognition and analysis of Cypriote ritual data', in Ioannides, G.C. (ed.), *Studies in Honour of Vassos Karageorghis* (Nicosia), 87–99.

Wilson, D.E. and Day, P.M. 2000. 'EMI chronology and social practice: pottery in the Early Palace Tests at Knossos', *Annual of the British School at Athens* 95, 21–63.

Xanthoudides, S. 1924. *The Vaulted Tombs of Mesara* (London).

Drinking with the Dead: Psychoactive Consumption in Cypriote Bronze Age Mortuary Ritual

David Collard, University of Nottingham

Previous considerations of the pottery assemblages found in Bronze Age Cypriote tombs have argued that rather than being grave offerings or personal possessions, the majority of artefacts are the residues of feasting by the living and that mortuary ritual was often an arena for social interaction (Manning 1998, 47; Steel 1998, 240; 2002, 109–110; 2004a, 168; Webb and Frankel 2008, 288). Furthermore, as bowls, jugs and juglets account for over 75 per cent of the pottery assemblage of all tombs for most of this period (Webb 1992, 89), it appears that the consumption of liquids, particularly alcohol, was a significant component of such activity. While other scholars have emphasized the important role of alcohol in generating conviviality in ritual contexts (Hamilakis 1998, 126; Manning 1993, 45; Sherratt 1997, 391; Steel 2002, 108; Webb and Frankel 2008, 290) corresponding evidence for the consumption of opium from Late Bronze Age tombs suggests that there may be other, as yet unconsidered, factors behind the consumption of such psychoactive substances during mortuary ritual. Instead of focusing on the role of such substances in relation to social interaction, this paper argues that it is their ability to produce profound spiritual experiences and psychological comfort for the individual that is of equal, if not greater importance.

Bronze Age Cypriote Mortuary Assemblages

At the start of the Bronze Age (*ca.* 2500 BC) a number of innovations are evident in Cypriote mortuary practice, including the use of rock-cut chamber tombs in formalized extramural cemeteries, multiple burial and possible secondary treatment of bodies, the reuse of tombs and significant increases in the wealth of grave-goods deposited, particularly metalwork and pottery (Keswani 2004, 37–82). Regarding the pottery, Manning (1993, 45) argues that the range of vessels deposited in Early Bronze Age tombs can be associated with the storing, pouring and serving of liquids and were used for the ceremonial consumption of exotic alcoholic drinks. Webb and Frankel (2008, 291) further suggest that the tulip bowls, jugs and deep bowls with spouts from this period can be associated with the consumption of beer as a component of funerary feasting. Later in the Early Bronze Age, the introduction of complex vessels comprised of multiple bowls and a reduction in jug size may indicate a shift from beer to wine (ibid., 292–293). Although this hypothesis is yet to be confirmed via organic residue analysis, iconographic evidence such as the winemaking scene on an Early Bronze Age Red Polished jug from Pygros (Flourentzos 1999), certainly suggests an association with wine and its production. Significant amounts of animal bone found in Early and Middle Bronze Age tombs also suggest that the sacrifice and consumption of adult cattle may have been a common component of these mortuary feasts (Keswani 2004, 67–68).

Webb and Frankel (2008, 292) argue that tomb elaboration and such promotional feasting were used to express status and negotiate access to resources within Bronze Age Cypriote society. The incorporation of these activities within mortuary ritual further suggests that ancestral relationships were central to the formation and legitimization of individual and sub-group identity (ibid., 292). Similarly, Steel (2002, 113) argues that the consumption of alcohol was explicitly associated with mortuary ritual in the Early and Middle Cypriote Bronze Ages, as a means for group legitimization via exclusive ritual centred on membership of ancestral groups.

In the Late Bronze Age (*ca.* 1650–1050 BCE) evidence for alcohol consumption in mortuary ritual continues in the form of tomb depositions of standardized, elaborate drinking services in Base Ring, White Slip and Bichrome Wheelmade wares, with mixing kraters as a centrepiece (Steel 1998, 290; 2002, 109). Bowls found inside kraters in tombs of this period (South 2008, 313; Steel 2004a, 174) suggest a common Cypriote practice of serving wine from these kraters. Considerable technical expertise seems to be invested in the manufacture of these drinking sets (Steel 1998, 290). Their use is also particularly evident in other contexts such as temples and monumental administrative buildings (South 2008, 313; Steel 2004a, 176–177). As the Late Bronze Age progressed, drinking sets in indigenous wares were replaced by more exotic Mycenaean-style sets (Steel 1998, 291), no doubt reflecting the increasing popularity of foreign imports. According to Steel (1998, 290), the increased elaboration of the drinking and serving vessels deposited in tombs suggests that ritual drinking was an important element of the Late Bronze Age practice of mortuary display.

This practice was not restricted to Cyprus, however, with elaborate drinking practices associated with mortuary ritual attested throughout the ancient Near East. For example, at Ugarit, located only 100 kilometres east of Cyprus, textual and archaeological evidence from the Late Bronze Age suggests the existence of ancestor veneration rituals involving the excess consumption of alcohol (Armstrong 1998, 92–93; McLaughlin 2001, 66; Pope 1972, 190–193). In particular, textual references to the *marzēah* (discussed further below) suggest the involvement of élites in a cult of the dead designed to legitimize and maintain their own authority (Steel 2002, 108; Armstrong 1998, 109; Carter 1995, 300–302). Notably, the strong economic and cultural ties evident between Cyprus and Ugarit include remarkable similarities in ceramic drinking sets (Steel 2004a, 174; 2004b, 185, n.142).

Concerning the Aegean, Hamilakis (1998, 128), has pointed out significant Bronze Age evidence for mortuary feasting and drinking ritual, including animal and plant remains, serving vessels and the construction of various delimited spaces to host such activity outside the tombs themselves. The prevalence of conical cups in Tholos tombs of the Cretan Mesara and drinking vessels such as *kylikes* in Mycenaean burials suggests

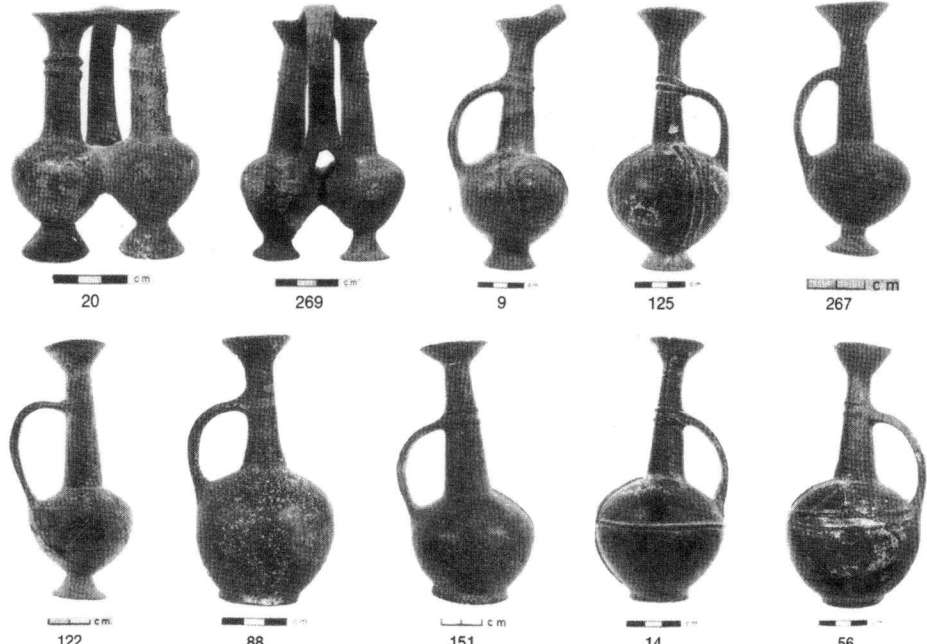

Figure 2.1. Base Ring juglets from Kazaphani-Ayios Andronikos Tomb 2 (after Nikolaou & Nikolaou 1989, Pl. XI).

an important role for the consumption of alcohol in the Aegean (ibid., 117). Cavanagh (1998, 106) has argued that the apparently intentional breaking of drinking vessels in the entrance of Mycenaean tombs may indicate a rite of separation as a component of mortuary ritual. Interestingly, Webb (1992, 88) makes a comparable suggestion for the Cypriote context, arguing that pottery used in funerary feasting was deposited in the appropriate tomb to prevent the efficacy of the ritual from being spoilt by its subsequent use for profane purposes.

Opium Consumption

Certain vessel types from Cypriote tombs indicate that, in addition to alcohol, other psychoactives, such as opium, were consumed as part of the mortuary ritual. Cypriote evidence for the consumption of opium, currently restricted to the Late Bronze Age, is best exemplified at the site of Kazaphani-Ayios Andronikos, located in north-central Cyprus. In Tomb 2 (Nikolaou and Nikolaou 1989) one of the two chambers contained 507 inventoried pots of which approximately 94 per cent can be associated with liquids. A similar situation can be seen in the other chamber, where 89 per cent of the 520 pots found can be associated with liquids. Of particular note, 100 Base Ring juglets (Fig. 2.1) were found in the first chamber and 128 were found in the second.

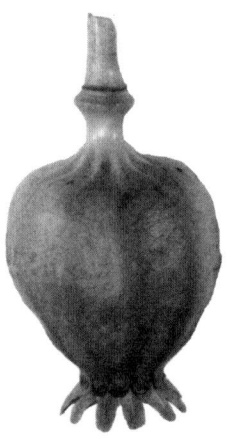 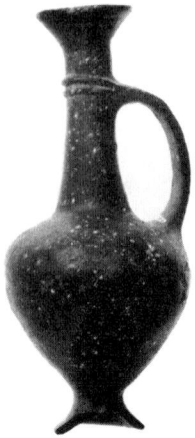

Figure 2.2. Opium poppy head compared with a Base Ring I juglet (after Merrillees 1962, Pl. XLII).

While this is easily the greatest number of Base Ring juglets found in a single tomb, this vessel is relatively common in other tombs, not only in Cyprus but also in Anatolia, the Levant and Egypt (Åström and Åström 1972, 143–161). Base Ring juglets have long been associated with opium by Merrillees (1962, 287–292) who argued that the shape and decoration of these juglets mimicked an opium poppy capsule (*Papaver somniferum*) incised to retrieve the psychoactive latex (Fig. 2.2), thereby advertising the vessel's contents as a liquid solution containing opium. This interpretation has recently been confirmed through the identification of opium alkaloid residues within both early and late examples (Koschel 1996, 161; Stacey pers. comm.). As the majority of the ceramic assemblages from Bronze Age Cypriote tombs appear to be associated with liquid consumption as a component of mortuary ritual, it seems feasible that significant quantities of opium were consumed in the ceremonies conducted in association with this particular tomb.

Altered States of Consciousness and Ritual

As there now appears to be evidence for the consumption of at least two different psychoactive substances during Bronze Age Cypriote mortuary ritual, it seems likely that it was in fact their psychoactive nature or, more precisely, their ability to induce altered states of consciousness that prompted their consumption in this context. As pointed out by the anthropologist Erika Bourguignon (1973, 3, 9–11), the experiential characteristics of altered states of consciousness commonly accord these phenomena an important role in the ritual practices of a wide range of ethnographically and historically documented cultures. These include feelings of intense emotion, changes

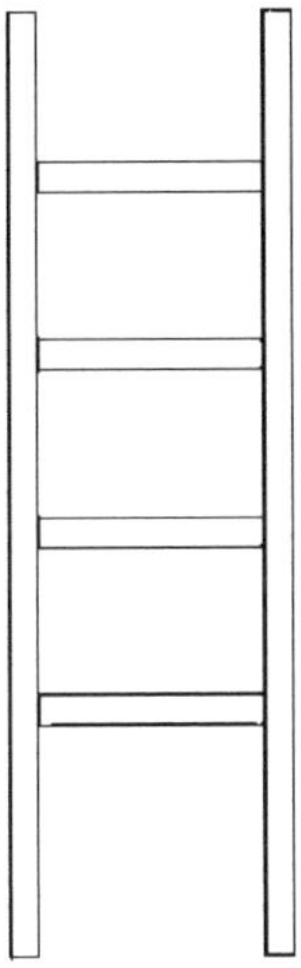

```
Religious institutions and
spiritual life

Social/political institutions

Subsistence-economics

Technology
```

Figure 2.3. Hawkes' 'Ladder of Inference' (D. Collard).

in body image, dissolution of boundaries between self and others – often interpreted as an experience of cosmic 'oneness', perceptual distortions and hallucinations and the ascription of increased meaning or significance to such experiences.

The cultural 'meaning' of such mental states can be approached by considering how they fit into a particular culture's religious or metaphysical beliefs. It has been observed that the worldviews of many cultures often involve a dualistic metaphysic, whereby a distinction is made between an 'everyday' world and a 'spirit' or 'other' world, where spiritual beings reside (Morris 2006, 313). In this context, entering an altered state of consciousness is commonly seen as a way to enter or interact with the supernatural world and its inhabitants (Bourguignon 1973, 3). This may particularly be the case in pre-modern contexts, where neuro-psychological explanations for altered states of consciousness were unavailable. Given that the beliefs behind mortuary practices commonly concern the soul and its journey to the world where ancestral spirits are thought to reside (Parker-Pearson 1999, 31), such metaphysical beliefs are clearly relevant to any consideration of mortuary ritual.

In light of these observations it may be possible to look beyond the socio-political aspects of mortuary feasting in Bronze Age Cyprus, to venture one rung further up Hawkes' ladder of inference (Hawkes 1954, 161–162) to the precarious heights of inference regarding religious beliefs (Fig. 2.3). How did the Bronze Age participants in mortuary rituals understand their experiences upon consuming alcohol or opium, particularly in relation to their metaphysical beliefs?

While it is notoriously difficult to read past beliefs from the remnants of rituals, it may be possible to approach nuanced inferences about such beliefs with the aid of ethnographic research and relevant iconographic and textual sources, at least in cases where there is also a significant amount of contextual archaeological data against which such evidence can be measured. Fortunately, a rich corpus of tomb assemblages, contemporary settlement data and residue analysis results can be combined with Late Bronze Age textual references to mortuary beliefs from nearby Ugarit to develop an understanding of the beliefs which lay behind the consumption of psychoactives during Bronze Age Cypriote mortuary ritual. Furthermore, as we know at least some of the specific substances consumed in this context, explicit consideration of the experiential characteristics of the alterations of consciousness they induce can further inform this interpretation.

Opium, for example, is commonly described to induce a feeling of overwhelming joy, bliss or euphoria and relax any tension and anxiety (Hayter 1968, 42; Rätsch 2005, 410). The sensation of flying or floating is common, with the combination of these two aspects commonly interpreted as an 'admission to paradise' (Hayter 1968, 42, 48). Visual hallucinations from opium consumption can exaggerate, multiply, colour or give fantastic shape to observed objects (Hayter 1968, 44). The possible aphrodisiac effects of opium consumption, however, are somewhat ambiguous (Meyer and Quenzer 2005, 248; Rätsch 2005, 410).

Concerning the experiential characteristics of alcohol consumption, low to moderate doses generally produce feelings of relaxation and cheerfulness, reduce inhibitions and slightly impair judgement and motor-skills (Meyer and Quenzer 2005, 244). At higher doses alcohol can induce lethargy, confusion and reduce memory, severely impair motor-skills and heighten a range of emotions including affection and aggression (Julien 2008, 107–109; Meyer and Quenzer 2005, 244). Extreme doses can cause a loss of bodily functions, unconsciousness and even death (Meyer and Quenzer 2005, 246).

Of particular relevance to the study of Bronze Age ritual, a number of these experiential characteristics correspond to those previously suggested to contribute to religious interpretations of altered states of consciousness. This suggests that alcohol- and opium-induced altered states of consciousness may have been interpreted as encounters with the spirit world. It is, therefore, unsurprising that the previously mentioned Ugaritic textual references to the *marzēah* suggest such an association.

The Marzēah

Throughout its 3000-year epigraphical history, the word *marzēah* has been consistently associated with an élite religious ritual involving the excessive consumption of alcohol in order to commune with ancestral spirits (Armstrong 1998, 93; Pope 1972, 190–193). It appears within nine Ugaritic texts dating to around 1200 BC, of which seven are legal documents and two are mythological texts (McLaughlin 2001, 11–26). One of these mythological texts contains a passage of particular relevance, translated as follows (ibid., 24–26):

> El sat, he assembled his drinking feast;
> El sat in his *marzēah*.

> El drank wine to satiety,
> New wine to drunkenness.
> El went to his house,
> He stumbled to his court.
> …..
> He floundered in his (own) faeces and urine,
> El collapsed like the dead,
> El was like those who descend to the underworld.

Clearly, El has consumed an extreme dose of alcohol. Due to the association between the *marzēah* and ancestor veneration ritual, the description of El collapsing 'like those who descend into the underworld' has been interpreted as a reference to El accessing the underworld via his drunkenness (Armstrong 1998, 104, 110). The *marzēah*, therefore, is identified as the ritual use of alcohol in order to bridge the gulf between the living and the dead (Armstrong 1998, 87). In this context, it is the ability of alcohol to provide an individual with access to the underworld that is emphasized, rather than its role in stimulating social interaction.

In light of this interpretation, therefore, it is possible that the widespread evidence for alcohol and opium consumption during Cypriote mortuary ritual reflects a similar attempt to access the world of the dead. Indeed, an association between Cypriote funerary rites and the *marzēah* has already been suggested by Steel (2002, 110), although this association is yet to be elaborated in any detail. In the context of either the primary or secondary burial of the dead, how might this possible attempt to access the underworld be interpreted?

Van Gennep (1960 [1908], 146–165), suggests that mortuary rituals can generally be considered as a three-stage rite of passage, with an initial stage involving separation from the world of the living, an intermediate liminal stage and a final stage involving post-liminal rites designed to ensure the incorporation of the deceased into the world of the dead. Without assuming that this exact ritual structure and underlying beliefs were also observed by the Bronze Age Cypriotes, the attempt to contact the underworld suggested in the consumption of psychoactives apparently coincides with the final interment of the body, suggesting a final, post-liminal stage of the ritual. As such, it is possible that the Bronze Age Cypriotes considered direct contact with the world of the dead to be a necessary part of their mortuary rites in order to ensure that the spirit of the deceased was finally accepted into this realm. Perhaps the deceased needed to be guided to the underworld by the living, perhaps the ancestors needed to be present at the feast or perhaps the living needed access to the underworld in order to pay appropriate homage to the deceased as a newly established ancestor.

As suggested by El's method of accessing the underworld during his *marzēah*, unconsciousness induced by large doses of alcohol would have produced experiential effects which could readily be interpreted by the subject as a temporary, but complete, descent to the underworld. The experiential characteristics of slightly lower doses of alcohol, such as lethargy, loss of motor-control and impairment of the senses, however, may have similarly been viewed as an intermediate contact with this realm, sufficient for a ritual function while being a far more practical state than unconsciousness. As even low doses of opium can induce sensations interpreted as contact with 'other-worlds', the addition of opium to the alcoholic beverage traditionally consumed may have been adopted in order to avoid the necessity of consuming large amounts of alcohol.

Conclusion

To conclude, I would like to turn back from the focus on past metaphysical beliefs to reconsider the importance of psychoactive substances from a psychological level. This is a theme intrinsically related to the role of such substances in the arena of social interaction and has previously been considered by Hamilakis (1998, 117) in relation to feasting in Bronze Age Aegean mortuary ritual: he argued that the emotions and senses stimulated by the consumption of food and drink in a mortuary context combine with those generated by the embodied experience of death to produce a powerful mnemonic device. The destruction and creation of memory is integral to mortuary ritual as the separation of the deceased from the world of the living involves erasing memory of them as a social player, thereby creating space for the renegotiation of social relationships between the living. As also argued by Steel (2008, 156) in the context of Cypriote mortuary ritual, the enhanced sensory participation on the part of the mourners promotes the creation of social memory and the renegotiation of individual and group identities.

While the disinhibiting properties of alcohol no doubt contributed to its important role in this creation of social memory, it may also have been the ability to suppress individual memory that gave alcohol and opium consumption such an important role in Cypriote mortuary ritual. Clearly, considerable emotional pain would have been associated with memories of the deceased for many of those involved in a mortuary ritual and the final interment is a context in which such raw emotion was likely to be felt most keenly. As such, suppressing memory, even if only temporarily, may have resulted in lessening the grief of the mourners, suggesting an important psychological benefit for the consumption of these particular psychoactives. This point is particularly emphasized by the following passage from Homer's *Odyssey*:

> Then Zeus's daughter Helen thought of something else.
> Into the mixing-bowl from which they drank their wine
> she slipped a drug, heart's-ease, dissolving anger,
> magic to make us all forget our pains …
> No one who drank it deeply, mulled in wine,
> could let a tear roll down his cheeks that day,
> not even if his mother should die, his father die,

> not even if right before his eyes some enemy brought down
> a brother or darling son with a sharp bronze blade.
>
> *Odyssey* 4, 243–251 (Fagles 1996, 131)

Given these arguments, the apparent popularity of the consumption of alcohol and opium during Bronze Age Cypriote mortuary ritual may relate to the ability of these substances to simultaneously reduce an individual's grief and erase their memories of the deceased, allowing the living to focus upon resuming social life without them. Consuming such substances, therefore, appears to have been important on the level of the individual, not only the social.

References

Armstrong, D.E. 1998. *Alcohol and Altered States in Ancestor Veneration Rituals of Zhou Dynasty China and Iron Age Palestine* (Lewinston, Queenston and Lampeter).

Åström, P. and Åström, L. 1972. *The Swedish Cyprus Expedition IV:1C. The Late Cypriote Bronze Age. Architecture and Pottery* (Lund).

Bourguignon, E. 1973. 'Introduction: a framework for the comparative study of altered states of consciousness', in Bourguignon, E. (ed.) *Religion, Altered States of Consciousness, and Social Change* (Columbus), 3–35.

Carter, J.B. 1995. 'Ancestor cult and the occasion of Homeric performance', in Carter, J.B. and Morris S.P. (eds) *The Ages of Homer, A Tribute to Emily Townsend Vermeule* (Austin), 285–312.

Cavanagh, W. 1998. 'Innovation, conservatism and variation in Mycenaean funerary ritual', in Branigan, K. (ed.) *Cemetery and Society in the Aegean Bronze Age* (Sheffield), 103–114.

Fagles, R. 1996. *Homer: The Odyssey* (Bath).

Flourentzos, P. 1999. 'A unique jug with a scenic composition from Pyrgos (Limassol District)', *Journal of Prehistoric Religion* 8, 5–10.

Hamilakis, Y. 1998. 'Eating the dead: mortuary feasting and the politics of memory in the Aegean Bronze Age societies', in Branigan, K. (ed.) *Cemetery and Society in the Aegean Bronze Age* (Sheffield), 115–132.

Hawkes, C. 1954. 'Archaeological theory and method: some suggestions from the Old World', *American Anthropologist* 56, 155–168.

Hayter, A. 1968. *Opium and the Romantic Imagination* (London).

Julien, R.M. 2008. *A Primer of Drug Action: A Comprehensive Guide to the Actions, Uses, and Side Effects of Psychoactive Drugs* (New York).

Keswani, P.S. 2004. *Mortuary Ritual and Society in Bronze Age Cyprus* (London).

Koschel, K. 1996. 'Opium alkaloids in a Cypriote Base Ring I Vessel (Bilbil) of the Middle Bronze Age from Egypt', *Ägypten und Levante* 6, 159–166.

McLaughlin, J.L. 2001. *The Marzeah in the Prophetic Literature, References and Allusions in Light of the Extra-Biblical Evidence* (Leiden).

Manning, S. 1993. 'Prestige, distinction, and competition: the anatomy of socioeconomic complexity in fourth to second millennium B.C.E.', *Bulletin of the American School of Oriental Research* 292, 35–58.

—— 1998. 'Changing pasts and socio-political cognition in Late Bronze Age Cyprus', *World Archaeology* 30(1), 39–58.

Merrillees, R.S. 1962. 'Opium trade in the Bronze Age Levant', *Antiquity* 36, 287–292.

Meyer, J.S. and Quenzer, L.F. 2005. *Psychopharmacology: Drugs, the Brain, and Behavior* (Sunderland Massachusetts).

Morris, B. 2006. *Religion and Anthropology: A Critical Introduction* (Cambridge).
Nikolaou, I. and Nikolaou, K. 1989. *Kazaphani: A Middle/Late Cypriot Tomb at Kazaphani-Ayios Andronikos: T.2A, B* (Nicosia).
Parker Pearson, M. 1999. *The Archaeology of Death and Burial* (Texas).
Pope, M.H. 1972. 'A divine banquet at Ugarit', in Efird, J.M. (ed.) *The Use of the Old Testament in the New and Other Essays. Studies in Honour of Franklin Stinespring* (Durham), 170–203.
Rätsch, C. 2005. *The Encyclopedia of Psychoactive Plants: Ethnopharmacology and its Applications* (Rochester).
Sherratt, A. 1997. 'Cups that cheered: the introduction of alcohol to Prehistoric Europe' in Sherratt, A. (ed.) *Economy and Society in Prehistoric Europe: Changing Perspectives*, (Princeton), 376–402.
South, A.K. 2008. 'Feasting in Cyprus: a view from Kalavasos', in Hitchcock, L.A., Laffineur, R. and Crowley, J. (eds) *DAIS, The Aegean Feast, Proceedings of the 12th International Aegean Conference, 25–29 March 2008, The University of Melbourne* (Liège), 309–315.
Steel, L. 1998. 'The social impact of Mycenaean imported pottery in Cyprus,' *The Annual of the British School at Athens* 93, 285–296.
—— 2002 'Wine, women and song: drinking ritual in Cyprus in the Late Bronze and Early Iron Ages', in Bolger, D. and Serwint, N. (eds) *Engendering Aphrodite: Women and Society in Ancient Cyprus* (Boston), 105–119.
—— 2004a. 'A goodly feast ... a cup of mellow wine: feasting in Bronze Age Cyprus', in Wright, J. C. (ed.) *The Mycenaean Feast* (Princeton), 161–180.
—— 2004b. *Cyprus Before History* (London).
van Gennep, A. 1960 [1908]. *The Rites of Passage* (Chicago).
Webb, J.M. 1992. 'Funerary ideology in Bronze Age Cyprus: toward the recognition and analysis of Cypriote ritual data', in Ioannides, A.G. (ed.) *Studies in Honour of Vassos Karageorghis* (Nicosia), 87–99.
—— and Frankel, D. 2008. 'Fine ware ceramics, consumption and commensality: mechanisms of horizontal and vertical integration in Early Bronze Age Cyprus', in Hitchcock, L.A., Laffineur, R. and Crowley, J. (ed.) *DAIS, The Aegean Feast, Proceedings of the 12th International Aegean Conference, 25–29 March 2008, The University of Melbourne* (Liège), 287–295.

Symbols of the Feasts: Élite Ideology and Feasting Practices in Early Iron Age Greece

Rachel Fox, University of Sheffield

The Early Iron Age (EIA – *ca.* 1100–700 BC) on the Greek mainland was a period of socio-political instability in comparison to the preceding palatial era, with small-scale village-based societies headed by leaders who drew on multiple spheres of authority to retain their positions. As power was both ascribed and achieved, it was necessary to demonstrate one's credentials for leadership in order to gain and preserve it. It is thus not coincidental that this era saw the revival of an élite 'package' that had been employed initially during the Early Mycenaean era, comprising references to specific activities that marked one out as belonging to the upper tiers of society. This 'package' consistently encompasses feasting, military activity, trade/travel, and ostentatious wealth. The *combination* of these factors, conspicuously expressed in prominent objects or scenarios, could successfully signal an individual as élite, as those of lower status would not be able to engage in these activities on an equivalent scale.

Each of the components of the élite 'package' was expressive of wealth and authority if manipulated correctly. Feasting demonstrated ownership of resources (livestock, arable products, manpower) and sufficient control to mobilize them. If large animals were expendable enough to be slaughtered, then they further emphasized the host's level of wealth. Martiality displayed possession of (expensive) weapons and access to leisure time in which to learn a skilled art form. Ability to wield weapons correctly could assist in acquiring authority through the threat of force. As for trade/travel, this expressed wealth through having the capital to embark upon such ventures, plus the mobilization of a ship and crew demonstrated authority. Additionally, travelling to foreign lands or the importation of foreign goods, in this particularly insecure period, appeared to ensure access to exotic realms, imbued with the mystique of distance (Helms 1988). When some or all of these factors were combined with ostentatious wealth, expressed through precious metal and imported items, they served to assert the owner's status.

I turn now to the material ways in which this élite 'package' was expressed throughout the EIA, specifically focusing on the element of feasting. I examine four areas in this paper that illustrate how feasting could operate as a part of the élite 'package': pictorial scenes on ceramic vessels, precious metal vessels, the interment of iron spits in warrior graves, and the presence of this élite ideology in the Homeric epics.

Pictorial Decoration

Pictorial decoration on ceramic vessels had been practised since LHIIIA (*ca.* 1300 BC); however, an increase in popularity and a change in subject matter can be noted in LHIIIC (*ca.* 1200–1100 BC) after the palaces' collapse. Unsurprisingly, iconography that was directly connected with the palaces, such as bull-jumping or boxing, completely disappeared in LHIIIC, while more timeless symbols of élite occupations increased and in some cases were newly portrayed (Vermeule and Karageorghis 1982; Thomatos 2006, 141). Examples of these include a sharp increase in chariot scenes (from 3.3 per cent of pictorial vases in LHIIIB to 26.3 per cent in LHIIIC, Vermeule and Karageorghis 1982), and an entirely new interest in foot soldiers and hunting activity. It is notable that these newly popular scenes focused on the sphere of militarism, one of the key components of the élite 'package'. Indeed, the images of chariots, infantry processions and animal hunts together comprise 46 per cent of the LHIIIC pictorial vessel corpus (Vermeule and Karageorghis 1982), thus indicating the significance that they held for those who commissioned or purchased the vessels. In the case of a small group of kraters from Kynos, East Lokris, sea battles are portrayed, thus referencing simultaneously the two élite activities of martiality and voyaging (cf. Dakoronia 2006a).

The élite subject matter of pictorial vessels was also deliberately conveyed to others. The most popular vessel for pictorial scenes was the krater, partly conditioned by the practical reason that it presented a large, relatively flat surface area. However, it may also be due to the fact that kraters acted as focal points during feasts or drinking rituals, due to their size and role in the formalized mixing process. Those invited to feasts would therefore have ample opportunities to view the vessels being used and to acknowledge the messages they bore – a combination of the wealth required to purchase large, fairly expensive vessels and of the élite scenes that were prominently displayed on them. Moreover, when the vessels were not in use, they remained eloquent by recalling to anyone who saw them the ability of the owner to partake in feasting activities and hence his capacity for an élite lifestyle. It may be wondered why feasting itself was extremely rarely portrayed on pictorial vessels, as the only certain images are a drinking ritual in the corner of a LHIIIC bowl from Tiryns and preparations for a funerary feast on an Attic LGI amphora when pictorial painting reappeared in the eighth century (Vermeule and Karageorghis 1982, 126, XI.19; New York 14.130.15, Boardman 1966). This may be due to the fact that feasting as an élite activity is already referenced in the form and use of the vessel and so it would have been over-compensation to portray commensal scenes as well. It was more effective when buying into an élite self-projection to reference multiple parts of the élite 'package' on one object.

After LHIIIC, pictorial decoration declined although large painted vessels still played an important role in defining status. It appears that the actual scenes were no longer what mattered but, in a process of symbolic reduction, the krater *vel sim.* could metonymically stand for an ideology of feasting activities and élite position in its own right. Probably the best-known example of this is the monumental krater from the tenth-century Toumba building at Lefkandi. While it bore a tree-of-life decoration, it was essentially non-figurative. Its extraordinary size and ornamentation, and its prominent location inside the nearly empty building, suggest that it was intended to make a statement of some sort. It has been proposed by Crielaard and Driessen (1994, 260–261) and Mazarakis Ainian (1997, 55–57) that it referenced the feasting the dead owner partook in during his lifetime, possibly even within that building, and I agree fully with this interpretation. This one vessel combines references to feasting, ownership of great wealth, and contact with the East in its orientalizing designs (Morris 2000, 228). It reveals that, by this point, it was not necessary to have explicit images of élite activity in order to express the owner's status. As a coda, the use of the Toumba krater as a form of *sema*, or grave-marker, foreshadows the later EIA practice of standing monumental vessels over the heads of tombs, particularly in the Kerameikos at Athens (Coldstream 1977, 33, 56, 61, 81). It is unclear whether the same symbolic meanings were current then, or whether the vessels were simply conveniently large enough to serve as appropriate markers, but it is possible that there was a retained memory of vessels signifying the owner's status.

Evidence for Metal Vessels

Another feasting-related method of expressing this ideological élite 'package' was through precious metal vessels, particularly when taken out of circulation and interred in a grave. The practice of burying metal vessels with the deceased had been current since the Shaft Grave period (MHIII/LHI, *ca.* 1600 BC) and the general symbolism of displaying one's wealth had hardly altered over the intervening centuries. In the EIA, it was a little less common than it had been during the Mycenaean era, possibly because there was less surplus wealth following the palaces' collapse. Hence, when metal vessels *were* interred, it can be assumed that the statements of wealth and social position being made were highly significant. In the LHIIIC cemetery at Perati, only two graves out of 249 yielded a metal vessel (Iakovides 1980, 99). The sheer rarity of metal vessels at this site may be compounded by the fact that the cemetery was used during a time of major socio-political change and hence surplus wealth may have been even more scarce. During the PG period (*ca.* 1050–900 BC), in the Toumba cemetery at Lefkandi, the proportion was slightly higher although still only a select few were privileged enough to be buried with metal vessels. Here they occurred in 11 graves out of 83 (Popham and Lemos 1996). In neither of these cemeteries is it clear by what justification one merited such a grave-good, as there is no obviously discernable pattern in the assemblages. It can only be said that they were not interred in the poorer percentile of the cemeteries, and therefore were not deemed as appropriate for low-status individuals. Significantly, several of the examples from the Toumba cemetery were near-eastern imports, including a bronze jug and two bronze bowls (graves T.47, T.55, T.70, Popham et al. 1989, 118–119; Morris 2000, 239). The idea of travel, a component of the élite 'package', is referenced here and again blended with feasting (in the vessel forms) and ostentatious wealth (in the precious metal) to create a web of symbolism in one grave-good. Trading for such valuable imports would have been the preserve of the élite, and being buried with the goods thus obtained would have declared this status by emphasizing access to faraway lands (Morris 2000, 235). Those who attended the funeral would have had the opportunity to view objects such as these vessels and would have received the intended messages that defined the deceased's actual and projected status.

Later than both Perati and Toumba was the MPG–EG (*ca.* 950–850 BC) cemetery at Atalante in East Lokris, which provides a capsule-type assemblage for examining the appearance of metal vessels (Dakoronia 2006b). Forty-three graves were excavated, of which only three contained a bronze bowl. Two were among the most well-furnished graves of the cemetery, in both cases part of a grave-good assemblage that contained weapons, multiple ceramic vessels and jewellery (Karagiorgos II and III, Dakoronia 2006b, 498). While perhaps not quite of the same tier as the other two tombs, the third bronze bowl was also found in a rich grave, alongside a wealth of jewellery (Dakoronia 2006b, 503). It can be seen that, while metal vessels were not automatically included in the wealthiest graves, they were not found in any tombs that were not notably rich; hence they could and did operate as status markers. One of the most well-appointed graves of the cemetery not only contained a bronze bowl but also a sceptre-like object (Karagiorgos II, Dakoronia 2006b, 498). The link cannot be made that this 'sceptre' equals kingship in the person of the deceased, but it is noteworthy that symbolic references to ruling (or a significant role in society) accompanied the interment of metal vessels, suggesting that they were regarded as appropriate for those of the highest social tiers.

Metal vessels were not simply interred in tombs and employed during feasting/drinking rituals, but could have further uses. First, they could serve as an urn for the deceased's ashes, such as the male individual in the Toumba building at Lefkandi who was buried inside a bronze amphora. Another, later, burial in the Toumba cemetery contained the ashes of the deceased inside a bronze cauldron (T.79B, Morris 2000, 249–250). While an amphora is a logical vessel in which to place ashes, due to the fact that it has a narrow mouth and can be sealed, a cauldron is less so and thus the choice of container may emphasize the vessel's symbolism. I would suggest that it was intended to create an association between the cremated individual and feasting that he performed during his lifetime, made more intimate by the fact that his ashes lay actually within a vessel that was inherently connected with commensality. Indeed, the assemblage in T.79B was constructed to reference the entire élite 'package': feasting in the cauldron, martiality in several weapons, travel through an antique Syrian seal, and wealth through the general richness of the grave-goods. While feasting was undoubtedly not the preserve of élite individuals such as this man, it can be observed how it was adopted as a way to express status that was as fundamental as the concepts of militarism and voyaging.

Secondly, metal vessels were dedicated in sanctuaries, particularly in the eighth century at the end of the EIA. These vessels were invariably tripod-cauldrons, massive and ostentatiously wealthy objects. It is notable that such dedications were often made at the largest and most frequented sanctuaries, such as Olympia, Isthmia and Delphi, where they would be observed by the greatest amount of people (Morgan 1990, 44–45; 1998, 85–86). While pious motivations were obviously intertwined with these dedications, such vessels would also be highly conspicuous and raise the dedicator's status, given that large numbers of visitors to the sanctuary could note his surplus wealth expended in the offering (Morgan 1990, 44–45). Again the arena of feasting was mobilized as a method of displaying social standing and wealth, albeit in a much more indirect manner. I turn now from vessels to iron spits, found throughout the EIA interred in only the most well-furnished graves.

Iron Spits

The practice of interring iron spits was current in mainland Greece from the later tenth century until the eighth century, when they became devalued and were abandoned as a method of highlighting élite status (Haarer 2001, 262–263). They were always interred in low numbers, as the highest quantity found in a single grave is 12 (Haarer 2001, 263). It has been argued by Courbin (1983) that they served as proto-currency, but I would prefer to follow Haarer's (2001, 247) interpretation that they were simply regarded as valuable objects, symbolically in their relation to feasting and actually by consisting of a large amount of iron. The majority of published spits come from graves in Argos, and it is from there that the best example comes, the so-called 'Panoply tomb' (grave 45, Courbin 1957; Coldstream 1977, 146; Haarer 2001, 266–267). This exceptionally wealthy grave contained 12 iron spits, plus a full set of armour, weapons and a pair of firedogs. The firedogs are in the form of warships and thus, together with the spits, the whole élite 'package' can be seen again in the references to travel, militarism, feasting and wealth. The firedogs showed signs of having been used (Courbin 1957, 378–379), and therefore they were not simply symbolic grave-goods, but attest the real practice of feasting during the life of the tomb's occupant. He appears to have been of sufficient wealth and status to have used commensality as a method of display both in life and after death.

As in the 'Panoply tomb', spits almost always accompany a wealth of grave-goods, particularly those of a military nature. Dickinson (2006, 158, 194) has drawn a connection between the interment of iron spits and warrior graves, and it is possible that spits did not simply make claims for the deceased to possess high social status but identified them with a particular élite subgroup, those renowned for martial valour and skill. It is perhaps not coincidental that the Homeric heroes' sole method of cooking was spit-roasting, attesting an ideological association between élite military status, the roasting of meat, and mythological conceptions of how heroes should behave. Spit-roasting was not a new cooking method in the EIA, as spit-supports have been discovered from the LHIIIB palace at Pylos, so instead this appears to be evidence for a new ideology surrounding it (*cf.* Sherratt 2004, 193). I wonder whether it is possible to trace here a means by which those of superior military status and wealth were presented in death as echoing the epic heroes, through having the ability to host impressive feasts. In a *milieu* where the mortuary sphere was a fundamental arena for displays and negotiations of status, this was a highly effective way of standing out from a myriad of other claims and would have been noted as conspicuously aggrandizing by funeral attendees.

Élite Ideology

There is not sufficient space here to detail my theoretical justification for using the Homeric epics as evidence but, in brief, I believe that the poems can serve as testaments of how people at the time of their eighth-century composition thought about certain social institutions and practices. Such a mental construction cannot be obtained from material evidence alone, and therefore broadens our perspective on how activities such as feasting were understood in the poet's own era and the recent past. There are glimpses in the poems of an inclusive participation in feasting; for example, the servants Eumaios and Philoitios dine with the aristocratic suitors in *Odyssey* 17 (256–260, 330–335). However, although it is clear that feasting was more inclusive in reality, the poems propagate an ideology by which it appears as the preserve of those of élite status. This accords closely with the archaeological record and the construction of the élite 'package', where feasting was presented to have a direct relationship with high social position, even though undoubtedly commensality was more inclusive. It appears that the poems provided documentation and justification of a belief that was shared by the élite and propagated in the ways that they manipulated material culture such as grave-goods.

In both epics, feasting is represented as a heroic activity. In the *Iliad* in particular, the heroes are portrayed feasting, while the ordinary soldiers eat for nutritional reasons only – a difference signalled by the words δεῖπνον (dinner) or δόρπον (supper), as opposed to δαίς (feast), which is used when the élite warriors dine. The inclusion of boys at feasts, such as Achilleus and Odysseus during their childhoods, implies that participation in commensality was based on ascribed status and therefore could be a marker of élite standing (*Il.* 9.486–489, *Od.* 16.442–444; Van Wees 1995, 175). Additionally, no one of non-élite status ever hosts a feast in either epic, with the exception of Eumaios, an episode required by the plot's exigencies and highly unusual in its vocabulary and components (Reese 1993, 161). While a closer study of the poems reveals glimpses of a more inclusive reality, generally this ideology is effectively maintained.

As mentioned, spit-roasting is the sole cooking method used in both epics. The only mention of any other method is of a boiling cauldron in a simile in *Iliad* 21 (362–364). Similes are the parts of oral epic that are most susceptible to change and therefore most likely to be contemporary, due to their purpose of explaining/enhancing an obscure image in terms that the listeners could comprehend. The whole description is rustic and non-epic in tone, and hence what we see here is the intrusion of a vernacular cooking method that varies sharply from the élite methods described elsewhere in detail. This is indeed the exception that proves the rule, as its inclusion in a contemporary-based simile indicates that (unsurprisingly) multiple cooking methods were practised in the eighth century, and the total focus on spit-roasting elsewhere suggests a deliberate strategy by the poet to present feasting as a wholly élite-centred activity. In addition, it can be noted that the heroes involve themselves in the cooking preparations, the best example being Achilleus when the embassy visits him (*Il.* 9.199–228). He does not leave the preparing of the feast to his servants, but fulfils all the required tasks and even serves the food. The conclusion can be drawn that the whole feasting process, from butchery to cooking to dining, was appropriate for heroes. In other words, feasting as an entirety had to have been emblematic of social status, or at least believed to be so, otherwise it would appear that those of the highest heroic status were prepared to abase themselves. As Achilleus had no reason to do this, given that he believed he was in the right at this point, his decision to cook and serve the meal must be due instead to the fact that feasting was an accepted method of demonstrating wealth, status and leadership qualities. Here it is worth remembering the inclusion of spits in warrior graves shortly before and around the period of the poems' composition, and the emphasis that they place on both commensality and food preparation accords closely with this scene from the *Iliad*. It is very likely that those buried with the iron spits were buying into the same ideology that was being promoted in the epics.

Conclusion
By examining multiple spheres of evidence such as ceramics, metal artefacts and poetic texts, it is possible to see the pervasiveness of the élite 'package'. Its ability to mark an individual as élite was achieved by incorporating a specific range of activities that were reliant upon high status to be performed to their full extent – feasting, martiality, trade/travel and ownership of ostentatious wealth – and by deliberately amalgamating two or more elements in one artefact or assemblage. These were then conspicuously presented as objects that multiple people would see (such as kraters) or at occasions where a crowd would gather (such as at a funeral). By concentrating on feasting in this paper, I have noted that a complex ideology surrounded this activity, whereby it was portrayed as being an élite practice even though that was almost certainly only part of the true situation. This concept was propagated through the deployment of commensal objects such as spits and vessels and through the method of poetic justification. It was therefore possible for leaders and would-be rulers of the EIA to capitalize upon this mindset and to employ feasting as an effective method for displaying and negotiating their authority.

References

Boardman, J. 1966. 'Attic geometric vase scenes, old and new', *Journal of Hellenic Studies* 86, 1–5.
Coldstream, J.N. 1977. *Geometric Greece* (London).
Courbin, P. 1957. 'Une tombe géométrique d'Argos', *Bulletin de Correspondance Hellénique* 81(1), 322–386.
—— 1983. 'Obéloi d'Argolide et d'Ailleurs', in Hägg, R. (ed.) *The Greek Renaissance of the Eighth Century BC: Tradition and Innovation* (Stockholm), 149–156.
Crielaard, J.P. and Driessen, J. 1994. 'The hero's home: some reflections on the building at Toumba, Lefkandi', *Topoi* 4, 251–270.
Dakoronia, F. 2006a. 'Mycenaean pictorial style at Kynos, East Lokris', in Rystedt, E. and B. Wells (eds), *Pictorial Pursuits: Figurative Painting on Mycenaean and Geometric Pottery* (Stockholm), 23–29.
—— 2006b. 'Early Iron Age élite burials in East Lokris', in Deger-Jalkotzy, S. and Lemos, I.S. (eds) *Ancient Greece: From the Mycenaean Palaces to the Age of Homer* (Edinburgh), 483–504.
Dickinson, O.T.P.K. 2006. *The Aegean from Bronze Age to Iron Age: Continuity and Change Between the Twelfth and Eighth Centuries BC* (London).
Haarer, P. 2001. 'Problematising the transition from Bronze to Iron', in Shortland, A.J. (ed.), *The Social Context of Technological Change: Egypt and the Near East, 1650–1550 BC* (Oxford), 255–273.
Hammond, M. 1987. *The Iliad* (London).
Helms, M.W. 1988. *Ulysses' Sail: An Ethnographic Odyssey of Power, Knowledge and Geographical Distance* (Princeton).
Iakovides, S. 1980. *Excavations of the Necropolis at Perati* (Los Angeles).
Lattimore, R. 1975. *The Odyssey of Homer* (New York).
Mazarakis Ainian, A.J. 1997. *From Rulers' Dwellings to Temples: Architecture, Religion and Society in Early Iron Age Greece (1100–700 B.C.) [Studies in Mediterranean Archaeology, vol. 121]* (Jonsered).
Morgan, C. 1990. *Athletes and Oracles: The Transformation of Olympia and Delphi in the Eighth Century BC* (Cambridge).
—— 1998. 'Ritual and society in the Early Iron Age Corinthia', in Hägg, R. (ed.) *Ancient Greek Cult Practice from the Archaeological Evidence* (Stockholm), 73–90.
Morris, I. 2000. *Archaeology as Cultural History: Words and Things in Iron Age Greece* (Oxford).
Popham, M.R., Calligas P.G. and Sackett, L.H. 1989. 'Further excavation of the Toumba Cemetery at Lefkandi, 1984 and 1986, a preliminary report', *Archaeological Reports* 35, 117–129.
Popham, M.R. and Lemos, I.S. 1996. *Lefkandi III: The Toumba Cemetery. The Excavations of 1981, 1984, 1986 and 1992–4: Plates* (Athens).
Reece, S. 1993. *The Stranger's Welcome: Oral Theory and the Aesthetics of the Homeric Hospitality Theme* (Ann Arbor).
Sherratt, S. 2004. 'Feasting in Homeric epic', in Wright, J.C. (ed.) *The Mycenaean Feast* (Princeton), 181–217.
Thomatos, M. 2006. *The Final Revival of the Aegean Bronze Age: A Case Study of the Argolid, Corinthia, Attica, Euboea, the Cyclades and the Dodecanese During LHIIIC Middle* (Oxford, BAR Inter. Ser. 1498).
Van Wees, H. 1995. 'Princes at dinner: social event and social structure in Homer', in Crielaard, J.P. (ed.) *Homeric Questions: Essays in Philology, Ancient History and Archaeology, Including the Papers of a Conference Organized by the Netherlands Institute at Athens (15 May 1993)* (Amsterdam), 147–182.
Vermeule, E. and Karageorghis, V. 1982. *Mycenaean Pictorial Vase Painting* (Cambridge, Mass.).

Intoxicating Drinks and Drunkards in Ancient Indian Art, Literature and Archaeology

Nitin Hadap and Shilpa Hadap, Deccan College, Pune

Today alcohol occupies an unusual position within Indian culture, its consumption being both permitted and proscribed across different sections of the population (Mohan and Sharma 1995, 128). However, in ancient India, the drinking of intoxicating beverages was very common practice for most people. Many liquors and intoxicating drinks are mentioned in the Vedic Literature (the body of Indian Sanskrit texts composed between 1500–500 BC) and both males and females are frequently depicted with drinking cups in ancient Indian art. Lovers enjoyed *Madhupāna* (the consumption of sweet mead-like beverages) in each other's company (Mahdihassan 1981, 223) and it seems that every occasion for celebration and social gathering, be it religious or secular, was turned into a drinking party. Although few other castes besides the Kśhtriya and Brāhmins are recorded as imbibing alcohol in historical texts, it is certain that almost the entire population was accustomed to drinking.

Given the apparent importance of drinking, there have been few major studies examining the role of intoxicating beverages in ancient Indian society; where research has been undertaken it has been restricted primarily to the historical evidence. This paper sets out to provide a more balanced impression of the situation by considering not only literary accounts but also iconographic and archaeological evidence for the consumption of intoxicating drinks. We should stress from the beginning that it is not our intention to provide a comprehensive review of drinking but rather to highlight the potential of studying foodways in ancient India and to show how they are directly connected to contemporary trends in regions to the west, in particular the Mediterranean.

Ancient Indian Literature: the Mirror of Contemporary Social Intoxication

Intoxicating drinks held an important position in religious as well as secular life in ancient India, indicated by the frequent references to liquor made in the Vedic Literature, such as the *Mahābhārata, Ṛgveda, Gāth-Saptaśatī, Purāṇas* and in the works of classical Sanskrit authors such as Kālidāsa. These texts reveal that intoxicating beverages were known by various names: the most common drinks were *Surā* and *Soma* (Mohan and Sharma 1995) as well as *Parisrut* (Mahdihassan 1981) but others include *Madya, Madirā, Āsava, Madhu, Surāsava, Gaudāsava, Madhāsava, Kṣudrā, Kailāvat Madhu, Phaljam Madhu, Madhumādhavi, Mādhavikā, Sauvīraka, Suvīraka, Sīdhu, Maireya, Vāruṇī, Madhuparka* and *Kadambari* (Joshi 1979a, 103; Lad 1979, 181).

Intoxicating Drinks and Drunkards

Surā was a kind of strong beer, prepared from grain (millet, barley or rice). It was drunk by all social groups, and was very popular with both the Kṣatriyas, the élite warrior class, and the peasant population (Mohan and Sharma 1995, 130; Sharma and Mohan 1999, 102). By contrast, the drinking of *Soma*, a spirit-like beverage, was regarded a high privilege and its consumption was restricted to nobles and saints, seers or holy men (Sharma and Mohan 1999, 102). Is said to have been prepared by pressing the sap from an as-yet unidentified plant (over a hundred botanical candidates have been proposed – see Nyberg 1995, 384) to obtain a juice that was mixed with water, milk or honey. In various ritual contexts it had a strong hallucinogenic effect and was understood to impart strength to warriors and the sick, eloquence to the poet, vision and insight to the priest, to cause fertility and even to grant *Amṛita* (immortality) to those who consumed it, as suggested in *Ṛgveda* 8.48.3:

> We have drunk *soma*; we have become free from death.
> We have gone to the light; we have found to the gods!
> What now can joylessness do to us?
> What truly, can the evil of mortality do?
> O you who are free from death?
>
> (Eliade 1987, 122–123).

Despite the many perceived benefits of *Surā* and *Soma*, excessive consumption was frequently associated with violent clashes. For example in the epic legend *Mahābhārata* the mythical characters Sundha and Upasunda killed each other in a drunken mace duel over the beautiful Tilottamā. The *Mahābhārata* also details the story of the Yadava clan who, maddened by wine, turned against one another, destroying the entire clan (Lad 1979, 181).

There is a clear association between warfare and alcohol, with soldiers drinking before battle, so that they might fight fearlessly, or afterwards to celebrate victory: for instance, according to *Brahmānda Purāṇa* and the *Brahma-vaivarta Purāṇa*, the hero Lord Balarāma drank deeply after defeating King Jarāsandha in the famous Chakra–Musala–Sangrāma war (Joshi 1979a, 2–3). But drinking was not the preserve of men; there is considerable literary evidence to suggest that women also regularly drank intoxicating beverages.

In the *Mahābhārata*, the princesses Draupadi and Subhadra, along with their female attendants, accompanied Kṛṣṇa and Arjuna to the bank of the river Yamunā where they abandoned themselves to drunken joy. Draupadi figures in another story of drunkenness when Queen Sudeṣṇā sent Draupadi to fetch wine from her brother Kīchak's palace – when Draupadi approached Kīchak with a jar, he promptly invited her to drink with him. The women most addicted to wine, however, appear to have been those from north-western India, from the kingdoms of Bāhlika and Madra. According to the *Mahābhārata*, they sang and danced in public places in drunken parties, threw off their clothes, and were even prepared to part with their jewellery (Lad 1979, 182).

Intoxicating Drinks and Drunkards

The writer Kālidāsa described the drinking of wine by women in his poems, suggesting that intoxication lends them a special charm (cited in Deo Prasad 1987, 94): for instance in his play *Mālavikāgnimitram* Queen Irāvatī comes to see the King having drunk wine, which was believed to give her added beauty. Vātsyāyana, a Hindu philosopher of the Vedic period, also records that women and queens had drinks in the palace on festival days such as Suvasantaka. This is supported by the sixth/seventh-century writer Daṇḍin, who mentioned that city women and wives of chiefs took drinks in the company of men and mixed freely with them during parties arranged by the King (Desai 1985, 175). For those of lower social status, drinking also took place in public houses known as *Pānagarṇi*, which were frequented by both men and women (Deo Prasad 1987, 94). However, these drinking houses gradually came to be viewed as harmful to the safety of a nation and the consumption of intoxicating beverages was equally condemned (Lad 1979, 181).

Strict rules against the drinking of wine by women were laid down in the *Smṛtis*, the body of Hindu scripture and customary law composed after the Vedas, some time around 500 BC. Prohibitions are made explicit in the *Manusmṛti* (Laws of Manu – *ca.* AD 200), which set out the religious, social and dietary obligations of different castes, and forbade Brāhmins from drinking liquor, or even discussing its sale (Schomp 2010, 25). The very fact that prohibitive legislation was created, suggests that the consumption of intoxicating beverages was rife, and indeed this is suggested by taxation records, such as the charter of Visnusena (AD 592), which makes reference to the taxes placed on wine and the distillation of spirits (Deo Prasad 1987, 95). Widespread drinking is also indicated by the iconographic record.

Iconographic Representation of Inebriates in Ancient India

Depictions of drunkards and drinking scenes are frequent in early historic Indian sculptures and paintings.

Kubera, the god of wealth, and his wife Bhadrā are commonly depicted holding wine cups in Gāndhāra and Kuśanā art, both cultures dating to the first to third centuries AD. In north India, during the Kuśanā period, Balarāma (brother of the great Indian god Lord Kṛṣṇa) is often depicted holding a flask of wine, but this type of image disappears in the Gupta period (mid-fourth to mid-seventh centuries AD). The Gupta period also brought a change in the depictions of Bhadrā, whose position seems usurped by the goddess Subhadrā (the sister of Lord Kṛṣṇa and Lord Balarāma). Subhadrā is depicted holding a *trishula* (a kind of trident), *khadga* (sword), wine cup and lotus in her hand and was worshipped by fraudsters, thieves, robbers and forest tribes (Joshi 1979b, 226).

Depictions of drunken women became particularly popular during the Kuśanā period thanks to the efforts of the Mathura school of sculpture (Varapande 2006, 56). Particularly fine examples of Mathura sculpture were discovered at the Buddhist *stupā* (mound-shaped monument for holding relics) at Sanghol, where a number of carved railing pillars depict women in a state of intoxication (Gupta 1985). One of the sculptures shows a girl holding both a flask of wine and a flute, a depiction that Varapande (2006, 60–64) argues is influenced by Greek traditions – in ancient Greece flute girls were in great demand as entertainers at drinking parties (ibid., 60).

Certainly there was considerable contact with the Mediterranean during the Kuśanā/Gāndhāra periods, which are frequently referred to as the Indo-Greek phase of Buddhist sculpture. Gāndhāra art seems to draw particularly upon the Roman tradition of Bacchus, and a number of sculptures depict Bacchanalian scenes (Joshi 1979b, 312). Contact with the Mediterranean world is also indicated by the styles of dress depicted in drinking scenes. For instance, at the cave site at Ajanta, a painting belonging to Vākāṭaka period (*ca.* AD 462–491) shows a number of foreign traders in drinking scenes, their costumes – conical caps, scarf, tunic and socks – and beards identifying them as Persians (Behl 1998). Another scene shows the Persian King Khusrau and his Queen Shirin, whose female attendant is holding narrow-necked vases (Dhavalikar 1999, 148–149). An amphora is seen in a painting in cave I at Ajanta, perhaps suggesting that Roman wine was imported up until the fifth century AD (ibid.); however, trade in wine is better understood through the examination of archaeological evidence – to which we now turn.

Archaeological Remains of Drinking Paraphernalia in Ancient India

Given the widespread iconographic evidence for drinking cups, their representation in the archaeological record is scarce. Some clay cups have been found in large quantities at north Indian sites dating to the Śuṅga (*ca.* 185–175 BC) and Kuśanā periods (mid-first to third centuries AD) and they have also been found in deposits dating to the Gupta period. However, the absence of drinking cups may relate to the materials from which they were manufactured: Kālidāsa refers to drinking cups (*droṇa*) made of betel leaves (*tāmbulānāṁ dalaih*), which seems likely given that wine cups made from banyan or palaśa leaves are in use even today (Dhavalikar 1965, 49).

Evidence for the production of intoxicating drinks, possibly the distillation of liquors such as *Soma*, has been claimed for two sites: Shaikhan Dheri in Charssada (first century BC to first century AD) and Taxila, now in Pakistan, which dates from about the third century BC to the fourth/fifth century AD. Both sites produced distinctive ceramic objects – globular pots, spouted cover-lids, terracotta tubes and spouted 'receiver' bowls – that Allchin (1979) has argued convincingly represent distillation paraphernalia, the earliest as yet discovered worldwide. Interestingly, the site of Taxila is famed for discoveries other than these local objects; it was also one of the first sites in India to claim the presence of imported Roman wine amphorae (Marshall 1951, 406). Subsequently, many more examples of Roman wine amphorae have been reported at sites across India including Arikamedu in Pondicheri; Ajabpura on the Machi river; Dwarka in Gujurat, and Nevasa Ahmednagar, confirming the strength of Indo-Mediterranean contact and trade in this period (Gaur et al. 2006; Gupta et al. 2001; Sagar 1992, 230; Wheeler et al. 1946).

Conclusion

This brief review of the historical, iconographic and archaeological evidence for the consumption of intoxicating beverages suggests that drinking was common practice in ancient India. Men and women, peasants and warriors, heroes and heroic gods – all were able to engage in drinking, often to excess. This tradition seems to have continued even into the time of the *Smṛitis* when intoxication became scorned and even prohibited, particularly for women. Amongst the Kuśanā and Gāndhāra cultures, for instance, iconographic and archaeological evidence suggests that drinking continued to be permissible for the upper classes and also amongst the Mediterranean traders who were responsible for importing wine.

At present, research into the role of intoxicating beverages in ancient India is in its infancy and a much more integrated approach to the evidence is required; however, we hope that this paper has highlighted the potential of such a line of enquiry.

Acknowledgements

We are thankful to Department of Archaeology, Nottingham University; Prof. Gouri Lad for her valuable guidance and to the authority, librarian and Staff of the Deccan Collage Pune. We are also thankful to Dr Pushpa Ranade, Director MNVTI, Pune, and Miss Pournima Chitale for their support and help.

References

Allchin, F.R. 1979. 'India: the ancient home of distillation?', *Man* 14(1), 55–63.
Behl, B. 1998. *The Ajanta Caves* (London).
Deo Prasad, K. 1987. *Taxation in Ancient India: From the Earliest Times up to the Guptas* (Delhi).
Desai, D. 1985. *Erotic Sculptures of India : A Socio-cultural Study* (New Delhi).
Dhavalikar, M.K. 1965. *Sanchi: A Cultural Study* (Pune).
—— 1999. *Historical Archaeology of India* (New Delhi).
Eliade, M. 1987. *The Encyclopaedia of Religion*, Volume 2 (London).
Gaur, A.S., Tripati, S. and Tripati, S. 2006. 'Evidence for Indo-Roman trade from Bet Dwarka Waters, west coast of India', *The International Journal of Nautical Archaeology* 35(1), 117–127.
Gupta, S., Williams, D. and Peacock, D. 2001. 'Dressel 2–4 amphorae and Roman trade with India: the evidence from Nevasa', *South Asian Studies* 17(1), 7–18.
Gupta, S.P. 1985. *Kushana Sculptures from Sanghol*, Volume 1 (New Delhi).
Joshi, N.P. 1979a. *Balarama* (New Delhi).
—— 1979b. *Bharatiya Murtiśastra* (Nagpur).
Lad, G. 1979. *Archaeology and the Mahābhārata*. Unpublished PhD thesis, University of Pune.

Madihassan, S. 1981. 'Parisrut: the earliest distilled liquor of Vedic times or of about 1500 B.C.', *Indian Journal of History of Social Science* 16(2), 223–229.

Marshall, J. 1951. *Taxial*, Volume 2 (Cambridge).

—— 1960. *The Buddhist art of Gandhara (Memoirs of the Department of Archaeology in Pakistan)*, Vol. I (Cambridge).

Mohan, D. and Sharma, H.K. 1995. 'Alcohol and culture in India', in Heath, D.B. (ed.) *International Handbook of Alcohol and Culture* (Westport), 128–141.

Nyberg, H. 1995. 'The problem of the Ayrans and the Soma: the botanical evidence', in Erdosy, G. (ed.) *The Indo-Ayrans of Ancient South Asia: Language, Material Culture and Ethnicity* (Berlin), 382–406.

Sagar, K.C. 1992. *Foreign Influence on Ancient India* (Delhi).

Schomp, V. 2010. *Ancient India* (New York).

Sharma, H.K. and Mohan, D. 1999. 'Changing sociocultural perspectives in alcohol consumption in India; A case study', in Peele, S. and Grant, M. (eds) *Alcohol and Pleasure: A Health Perspective* (Philadelphia), 101–120.

Varapande, M.L. 2006. *Women in Indian Sculpture* (Delhi).

Wheeler, M., Ghosh, A. and Deva, K. 1946. 'Arikamedu: An Indo-Roman trading-station on the east coast of India', *Ancient India* 2, 17–124.

A New Renaissance Medical Controversy: Sixteenth-Century Polemics About Cold-Drinking

Justo Hernández, University of La Laguna, Spain

From a general perspective Galenism – the medical body of knowledge articulated by the Greek physician Galen (129–211/216) and completed by his followers – seems to be a homogeneous doctrinal corpus, particularly concerning pathology. In medieval Europe Galenism was accepted unquestioningly as the medical orthodoxy but the Renaissance, with its characteristic intellectual autonomy, brought about a reappraisal of Greek medicine. Renaissance Galenism has rightly been considered disputatious, with scholars of the time questioning received wisdom and encouraging dissent from mainstream medical practices, such as blood-letting. Even marginal tenets were open to discussion, particularly among minor authors. This paper will explore a particular controversy of this period by examining a series of Spanish medical texts written between 1555 and 1576. The texts relate to dietetics and, in particular, to the issue of cold-drinking, the focus of this paper.

The Issue of Cold-Drinking

Cold-drinking means, simply, drinking cold fluids. It seems wise to begin by clarifying why cold-drinking became an important issue for Renaissance medicine. The answer can be found by examining the central medical theory and practice of Galenism: the belief that health was based on achieving the proper complexion (i.e. temperament) of the human body. A healthy temperament for men was deemed to be warm and dry, whereas for women the temperament should be cold and moist. It is important to note that the body's temperament could be balanced or unbalanced by the effect of drinks and/or foods consumed. Following classical Greek medicine, medieval masters condemned cold-drinking on the basis that it would cool the naturally warm temperament of men and be dangerously cooling for women, who were already cold and moist (Albala 2002, 48–52). Magninus (Ms. 873, 6r) wrote that very cold water from snow and ice should be avoided lest the functions of the organs be fatally altered, as was observed in 1506 when the King of Castile, Philip I, took an excessively cold drink while sweating profusely from a ball game – this brought on a fever and he died a few days later (Suárez 2004, 407). It was claimed that the King's fate was sealed not only by the cold temperature of the lethal beverage but also by the fact that he drunk it all at once – it was fatal because his body was not used to such cold.

The Sixteenth-Century Debate

References to cold-drinking are found in two important medical books published in the mid-sixteenth century. They may be considered the starting-point of a debate which would divide doctors and society alike: the question being whether cold-drinking was healthy or not.

The first belongs to the Spanish version of Dioscorides' *Materia Medica* (1555) by Andrés Laguna (1510–1559). According to this (Fig. 5.1), the drinking of cold water carried a high risk of suffocation caused by cardiac malfunction from the cooling of the heart, an organ characterized by its naturally hot temperament (Laguna 1555, 596). It was the sudden contact of the cold drink with the heart that was said to prevent the body from adapting to the new temperament, which could be then fatal. Laguna (1555, 511) stated that wines cooled with ice, snow or saltpetre destroyed the teeth, reduced natural heat and gradually led to many 'cold diseases' (i.e. those that had, or were caused by, a cold temperament) such as stroke, asthma and oedemas. He believed that these diseases were prevalent amongst people who habitually drank cold beverages, and he talked disapprovingly of the north-European fashion for cold-drinking which was then adopted in Spain by ordinary people, noblemen, princes, priests and bishops (Laguna 1555, 504). It should be remarked that Laguna's criticisms concerning the noxiousness of this habit were directed particularly at the highest clerical dignitaries – or those who were prone to cold-drinking at the time – a period, it should be noted, that followed hard on the first emergence of Protestant reform in northern Europe and the Council of Trent in the south.

The second key source is *Liber de Arte Medendi* [Book of the Art of Medicine] by Cristóbal de Vega (1510–1573), finished in 1557 and published in 1564. Here, de Vega clearly condemns drinking wine cooled with snow or ice, explaining that it is a particularly dangerous practice because people drink it both in summer and in winter. He compares the habit of cold-drinking, common amongst noblemen, to a pernicious plague that ravaged first the Germans, later the Flemish and the French, and finally the Spanish, once their traditional sobriety had disappeared (de Vega 1564, 227).

The Only Manuscript on Cold-Drinking

There is a brief unpublished manuscript that was written in 1569 by Luis de Toro (*ca.* 1530–?, *fl.* 1574), entitled *Discursos o Consyderaciones Sobre la Materia de Enfriar la Bebida* [Discourses or Considerations on the Matter of Cooling Beverages]. It is a three-person exchange of ideas between Águila, a physician in favour of cold-drinking, Sylva, who is against it, and Claudio who acts as chair-person. The prologue reveals that de Toro is, in fact, Sylva, as he considers cold-drinking a vice related to gluttony (de Toro 1991, 229).

Águila contends that cold-drinking is as natural as the desire to satisfy one's thirst and refresh the throat. Indeed, cold-drinking has existed in every country of the world (de Toro 1991, 234–235). In reply to questioning by Claudio, he maintains that Galen

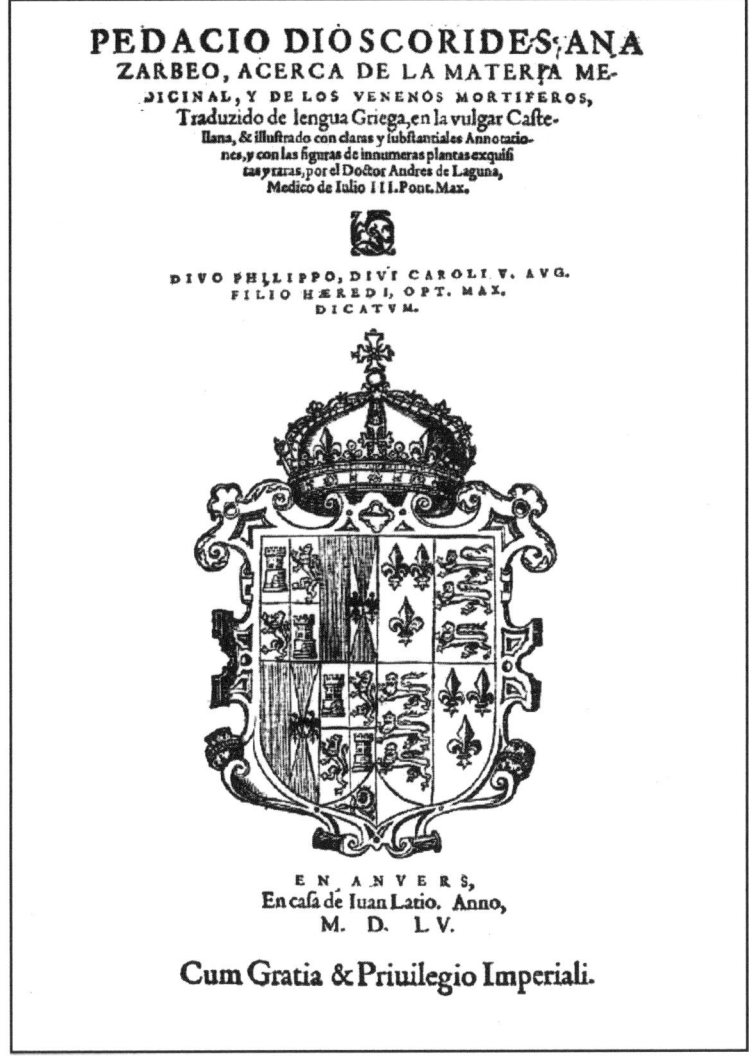

Figure 5.1. Title page of Pedacio Dioscórides... *edited and translated by Andrés Laguna (Biblioteca Histórica 'Marqués de Valdecilla', Madrid).*

refers to these habits among Romans in many of his works (de Toro 1991, 242). Águila's strongest claim, however, is that Charles V used to cool his wine, water and beer with snow, as did Philip II somewhat later (de Toro 1991, 244).

Sylva retorts that cold-drinking had become fashionable over the last twenty or thirty years to the detriment of human health. He emphasizes the harm caused by this pernicious habit and complains about its spread to all levels of society (de Toro 1991, 244–245). It should be pointed out here that de Toro provides us with an approximate date for the adoption of this custom, which he places around 1539, when the Imperial Age under Charles V gained momentum. To refute Águila's claim, Sylva points out that he has seen many people, from a variety of social backgrounds, die from cold-drinking, even noblemen and bishops (de Toro 1991, 262). He does, however, mention an exception: that moderate cold-drinking is permissible in summer and in hot areas for men, though not for women as their temperament is too humid and cold (de Toro 1991, 276). With regard to men, it is suggested that cold-drinking may be allowed provided they are between 15 and 45 years of age, when the beverage would balance their temperament. Under 15 years their temperament was thought not warm and dry enough, and after 45 it was considered too cold and dry (de Toro 1991, 276–277).

An Early Defence of Cold-Drinking

Francisco Franco's (ca. 1515 – post 1569) *Tratado de la Nieve y del uso della* [Treatise on Snow and its Use] was published in 1569. It is a 15-page booklet, addressed to a nobleman from Seville, which presents Franco's opinions about cold-drinking (Fig. 5.2). The author explains in the *epistola nuncupatoria* that there is much dispute on the topic (Franco 1984, 51). Nonetheless, he defends drinking beverages cooled by snow on condition that the snow is not actually placed in the glass but rather packed round the vessel (Franco 1984, 53). Since Franco is writing about Seville, he insists that cold-drinking by men is not only healthy but necessary, especially during the summer when the heat is extreme (Franco 1984, 54). In relation to the age of men or women who could indulge in cold-drinking he suggests that it should be limited to people from 14 to 60 years of age. It is not allowed for children and elderly people, whose faculties are considered weak, particularly in childhood when the nerves were considered to be thin and fragile (Franco 1984, 63).

Concerning women, Franco concedes that they can drink cold beverages to their benefit unless they suffer from hysteria in the classical Greek sense, that is, from disturbances of the womb (Franco 1984, 68). According to Franco, healthy women living in hot climates were allowed to drink cold beverages. Finally, Franco refers to the strongest claim for cold-drinking: its use at the Spanish court. He states that the King's doctors allowed him to have cold drinks and therefore the practice cannot be regarded as unhealthy (Franco 1984, 74).

An Appendix to a Book on American *materia medica*

Nicolás Monardes (ca. 1493–1588) wrote a book entitled *Libro que trata de la nieve...* [Book Dealing with Snow], a 47-page treatise that was printed as an addition to his important work on the American *materia medica* (Fig. 5.3). In the *epistola nuncupatoria*, dedicated to a prestigious physician, the author states that he wants to find out whether or not drinking cold beverages is healthy, as it is such a controversial issue. Moreover, he affirms that the adoption of this habit was related to gluttony, although it seems clear that he approves of, or at least tolerates the vice (Monardes 1574, iv).

Sixteenth-Century Polemics About Cold-Drinking

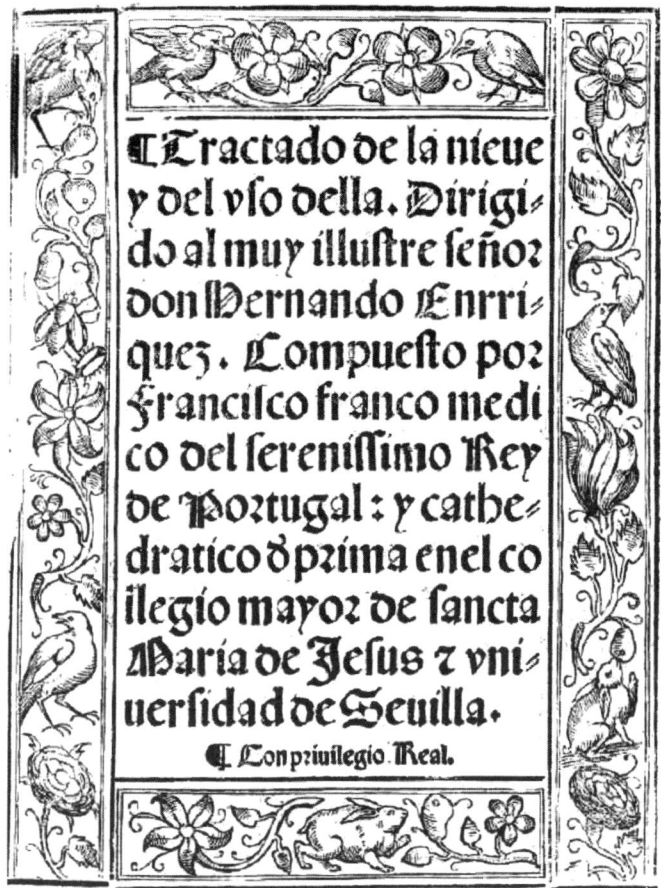

Figure 5.2. Title page of Tractado de la nieve... *by Francisco Franco (Biblioteca Histórica 'Marqués de Valdecilla', Madrid).*

Monardes stresses that the best property of snow is its ability to cool drinks, to this end it is employed all over the world (Monardes 1574, 9r–9v). He says that snow water, by its very nature, is similar to rain water and thus should not be condemned. It is totally harmless, is indeed what is found in most rivers and is drunk thoughout Spain and Germany, and even more widely in America (Monardes 1574, 24v–25r).

By contrast to the authors that preceded him, he claims that rather than unbalancing the temperament, cold-drinking actually tempers the liver, attenuates heat, excites the appetite and quenches thirst (Monardes 1574, 29r–29v). He is astonished that in Seville there are no facilities to conserve snow for cooling beverages, given that cold-drinking is necessary due to the great heat (Monardes 1574, 28r–28v).

Along with other authors, he endorses cooling with snow as the best way to cool beverages but condemns the snow itself, except for those who need it as a medicine, because it gives rise to many diseases (Monardes 1574, 32v–33r, 34r–34v). Concerning age-related cold-drinking, Monardes follows classical doctrine to recommend that it should not be permitted to children or elderly people (Monardes 1574, 35v).

A Medical Book About Water

In 1576 Alonso Díez Daza published the only medical book dealing with water in sixteenth-century Spain. In the second book of *Libro de los Provechos y Dannos que Provienen con la Sola Bebida del Agua...* [Book on the Benefits and Harms from Just

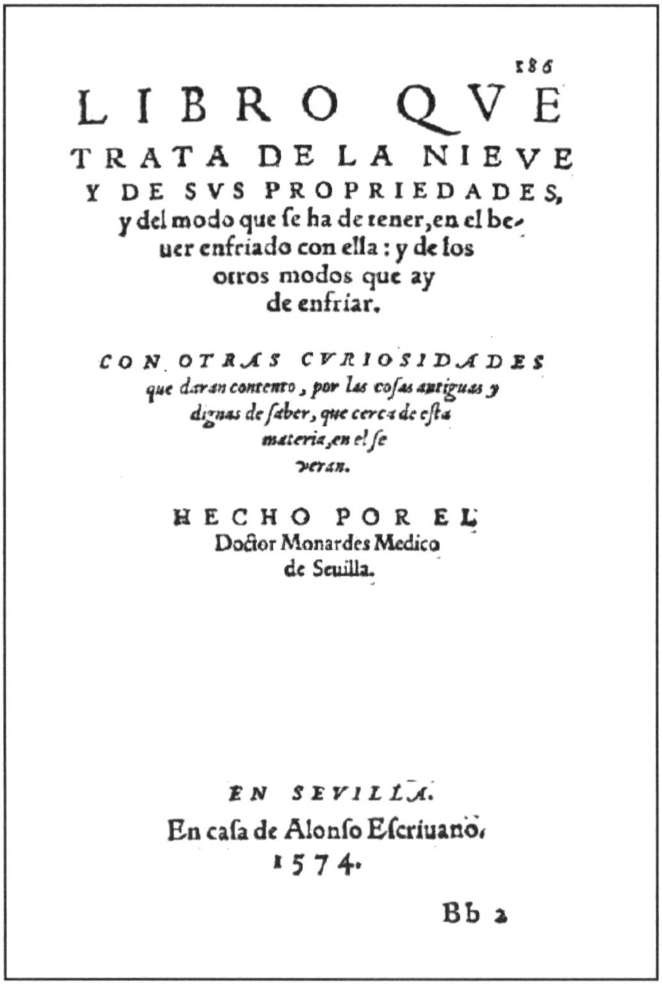

186

LIBRO QVE
TRATA DE LA NIEVE
Y DE SVS PROPRIEDADES,
y del modo que ſe ha de tener, en el be-
uer enfriado con ella: y de los
otros modos que ay
de enfriar.

CON OTRAS CVRIOSIDADES
que daran contento, por las coſas antiguas y
dignas de ſaber, que cerca de eſta
materia, en el ſe
veran.

HECHO POR EL
Doctor Monardes Medico
de Seuilla.

EN SEVILLA.
En caſa de Alonſo Eſcriuano.
1574.

Bb 2

Figure 5.3. Title page of Libro que trata de la nieve... *by Nicolás Monardes (Biblioteca Histórica 'Marqués de Valdecilla', Madrid).*

Sixteenth-Century Polemics About Cold-Drinking

Drinking Water] he sought to show the best way to drink cooled water so as to make it harmless to the body.

With regard to waters from snow and ice, Díez Daza writes that they are pernicious by reason of their heaviness and claims they can harm the liver. He finds no explanation for some physicians endorsing these forms of water (Díez Daza 1576, 47v–48r), and suggests that it is preferable to drink fresh, pure water (Díez Daza 1576, 56v–57r). Díez Daza establishes five conditions which should be fulfilled in order to drink cold water safely: 1) to be in the habit of doing it; 2) not be an elderly person; 3) to take cold drinks only in summertime; 4) to have a warm temperament; and 5) to have healthy bowels (Díez Daza 1576, 70v–71r).

At the end of his book, and taking Galen's observations into account, Díez Daza proposes a method whereby cold or cooled water may be consumed without harm: before cooling good-quality water with snow, it should be boiled. In this way, no harm would come in summer to persons of any age or temperament (Díez Daza 1576, 122v–123r).

The Treatise on Cold-Drinking

In 1576 Françesc Micó (1528–*post* 1576) published the most complete and most authoritative treatise on cold-drinking: the 145-page book *Alivio de Sedientos...* [Relief of Thirsty Persons]. In this volume Micó asserts that the most natural way of drinking is to consume cold water, but that gluttony has corrupted this practice (Micó 1576, 11r–11v). He states that cold-drinking is healthy, especially in hot and populous places or towns (Micó 1576, 17r–17v). He admits that denizens of such places, as well as violent individuals, can drink without risk thanks to their excessively hot temperaments.

As with scholars before him, Micó (1576, 23v–24r) suggests that the best way of cooling beverages is by placing the snow close to, but not in the cup which contains the liquid – to mix in the snow could be harmful to organs such as the kidneys (Micó 1576, 50r). He offers additional advice about the kinds of cups that should be used, recommending glass or silver vessels (Micó 1576, 56v). Where he breaks with tradition is to suggest that the benefits of cold-drinking are infinite – with the capacity to heal many diseases (Micó 1576, 78v–79r). He does not understand why physicians speak against the practice (Micó 1576, 88r–88v) and argues that the variations cold-drinking produces in the temperament of healthy people are only minor. Micó remains conservative in his advice on age and gender, recommending against the consumption of cold drinks by weak individuals such as children, the elderly, women, and persons suffering from diseases of the stomach or from diseases caused by cold temperaments (Micó 1576, 97r).

Micó reiterates the common claim that cold-drinking was widespread – from Italy to Flanders, Germany, France, Spain, Turkey and elsewhere – and that people from different strata of society, from princes to peasants, share the habit (Micó 1576, 125v–126r). However, rather than condemning the practice, Micó concludes that cold-drinking is perfectly healthy.

Sixteenth-Century Polemics About Cold-Drinking

Conclusion

Authors such as Andrés Laguna, Cristóbal de Vega and Luis de Toro considered cold-drinking a pestilence or an epidemic of gluttony. This view gradually changed and the habit was then deemed a delight permissible to kings, noblemen and ordinary people. Medical admonitions were in vain. In this controversy, which began in mid-sixteenth century, the battle was easily won by those physicians who endorsed cold-drinking, because the only book which could have had an impact both on the medical and lay opinion, Luis de Toro's dialogue, was never printed. Nicolás Monardes' idea of attaching his booklet on snow to his great work *Historia medicinal de las cosas que se traen de nuestras Indias Occidentales* was a good one, giving it the chance to achieve a diffusion not enjoyed by any other text on the topic.

All these texts provide interesting information about past attitudes to health and well-being, and demonstrate how transient, even contradictory, medical advice can be. It is difficult to comprehend how the act of cold-drinking – a practice undertaken today without thought – can have inspired so much debate. But this serves to remind us just how important were food and drink in the past.

References

Albala, K. 2002. *Eating Right in the Renaissance* (Berkeley).
de Toro, L. (ed. Sanz Hermida, J.) 1991. *Discursos o Consyderaciones Sobre la Materia de enfriar la bevida* (Salamanca).
de Vega, C. 1564. *Liber de Arte Medendi. Cum Indice Locupletissimo* (Lyons).
Díez Daza, A. 1576. *Libro de los Provechos y Dannos que Provienen con la Sola Bebida del Agua* (Seville).
Franco, F. (ed. Santonja, G.) 1984. *Tractado de la Nieve y del uso Della* (Madrid).
Laguna, A. 1555. *Pedacio Discórides… Acerca de la Materia Medicinal* (Antwerp).
Magninus Mediolanensis. *Regimen Sanitatis ad Dominum Antonium de Flisco*. Ms. Paris, Bibliothèque d'Arsenal, 873 (fifteenth century), 1r–34r.
Micó, F. 1576. *Alivio de los Sedientos* (Barcelona).
Monardes, N. 1571. *Libro que Trata de la Nieve, y de sus Propiedades* (Seville).
Suárez, L. 2004. *Fernando el Católico* (Barcelona).

Living and Eating in Coastal Brazil during Prehistory

*Mercedes Okumura and Sabine Eggers,
Universidade de São Paulo*

During the second half of the Holocene, almost the entire Brazilian coast was densely colonized by shellmound-building groups (Fig. 5.1a and d). Around 1000 shellmounds have been recorded by the Brazilian Institute for the Historic and Artistic Heritage (IPHAN) but this is certainly an under-representation of what once existed (Gaspar 1998, 593). Shellmounds are found from the state of Rio Grande do Sul to Bahia and, whilst they are sparse in the north and north-east, they are particularly numerous in the south (from Rio de Janeiro to Santa Catarina state), which has been the focus of most research, including this paper.

With a few exceptions, the shellmounds of southern Brazil date to between 6500 and 800 BP, with a peak between 5000 and 3000 BP (Lima 1999–2000, 272). Physically, shellmounds can be huge, reaching 30 metres in height and several hundred metres in diameter, as is often found in the state of Santa Catarina (Fig. 6.1c). The large size and long duration of these sites suggest considerable human adaptation to the coastal environment.

The Brazilian word for shellmounds is *sambaqui*, a Tupi word deriving from *tamba*, meaning mollusk, and *ki*, meaning accumulation (Prous 1991, 204). Brazilian shellmounds have been known since the sixteenth-century when Portuguese colonizers explored them as a commercial source of lime (Lima 1999–2000, 286). However, it was only in the nineteenth century that shellmounds began to be investigated by naturalists and amateurs who debated whether they were the result of natural or anthropic actions: the Brazilian scientific community finally reached a consensus that the shellmounds were intentionally built in the 1960s (Lima 1999–2000, 287). By the late 1970s Chmyz (1976, 12) was able to define shellmounds as 'artificial mounds of stratified shells, fish bones …, in which the proportion of shells usually is higher than 70 per cent in relation to the other elements'. This highlights the fact that shellmounds contain materials other than shell and, of these materials, pottery is perhaps the most intensely studied cultural marker.

Shellmound pottery is one of the few well-established chronological markers for the prehistoric Brazilian coast (Lima 1999–2000, 285) and its arrival seems to coincide with considerable changes in the lifestyle of these coastal groups (Lima 1999–2000, 285). The earliest pottery evidence on Brazilian coastal sites dates from 1,000 BP. It is usually divided into two groups, one in the states of Rio de Janeiro and Espirito Santo to the

Living and Eating in Coastal Brazil during Prehistory

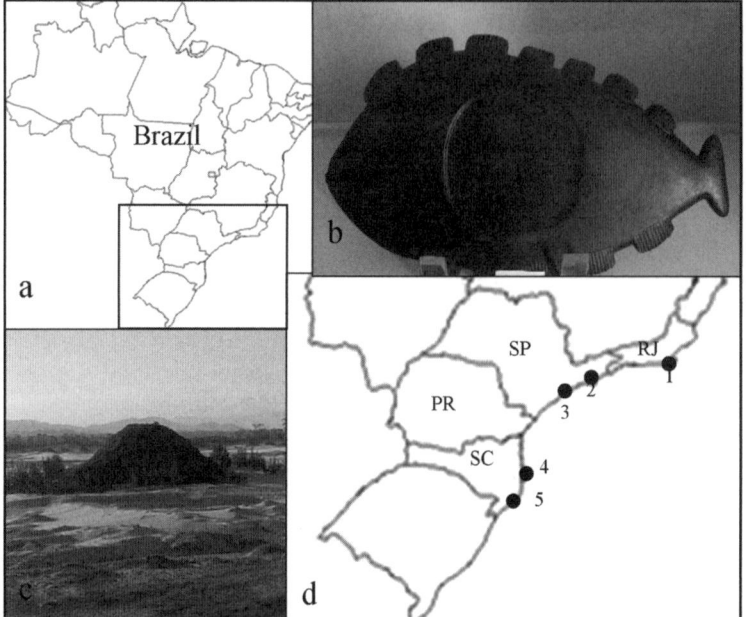

Figure 6.1. a) map of Brazil presenting the area shown in greater detail in d; b) polished stone figurine representing fish; c) shellmound site; d) detail of map showing states (RJ: Rio de Janeiro; SP: Sao Paulo; PR: Parana; SC: Santa Catarina) and location of sites mentioned in the article (1: Beirada; 2: Tenorio; 3: Piacaguera; 4: Forte Marechal Luz, Enseada I, Itacoara, Ilha de Espinheiros II, Morro do Ouro, and Rio Comprido; 5: Cabecuda and Jabuticabeira II).

immediate north, and the other on the coasts of the states of Santa Catarina and Paraná. Both traditions may have originated inland and spread subsequently to the coast. The arrival of groups with pottery must have accelerated the end of the shellmound societies, either through extinction or absorption. It is interesting to note that, at least in the northern region of Santa Catarina, the ceramic levels are associated with the arrival of a new biological group (defined in terms of cranial morphology) distinct from the pre-ceramic one that built the shellmounds (Neves 1988, 140; Okumura 2008, 296).

In the past, shellmounds were viewed as the product of small, nomadic mollusc-eating groups who sought to construct dry platforms in flood-prone areas. However, this view seems too simplistic. Certainly the mounds cannot be explained in terms of flood-protection because they are often much higher than would be necessary; furthermore, many were built in areas not liable to inundation (Gaspar 1998, 597). Instead it would seem that shellmounds acted as funerary structures (human burials have been found in most of them – Gaspar 1998, 597) as well as places of habitation (based on the presence of dwellings and their associated artefacts – Gaspar 1998, 602). This suggests some sedentarism, a hypothesis that has been confirmed indirectly by studies of the human remains which exhibit high levels of infectious diseases – these tend to thrive best in sedentary groups (Okumura and Eggers 2005, 277). In addition, the skeletal remains displayed little evidence of trauma and this, together with the fact that several neighbouring shellmounds were in use at the same time, indicates resource abundance: in other words, a situation conducive to supporting sedentary occupation (Okumura and Eggers 2005, 266; De Blasis et al. 2007, 58).

Today, shellmound builders are considered to have been sedentary people with a relatively complex social organization (De Blasis et al. 1998, 102; Gaspar et al., 2008, 323). This paper seeks to advance our understanding of their lifestyle and subsistence practices by drawing together evidence from a wide range of studies: zooarchaeology, human remains analysis (including palaeopathology and isotopic studies), palaeobotany, anthracology, phytolith and starch analysis, as well as investigations of artefact types.

Zooarchaeology

As the major constituent of shellmounds, debate has surrounded the archaeological significance of the shellfish themselves. Even when the anthropic nature of shellmounds was finally established, scholars believed that they were simply the food-remains of highly mobile shellfish-eating populations (Lima 1999–2000, 287). Later, zooarchaeological studies showed that, although very conspicuous in these sites, shellfish was only a secondary source of calories and that diet was based primarily on fish, with birds and rodents making a minor contribution at sites such as Jabuticabeira II (Figuti 1993, 71; Kneip 1994, 62; Klokler 2001, 110, 122).

Today, the very idea that the shellfish were food is being challenged; several scholars argue that they were more probably used as construction material (De Masi 2001, 7; Gaspar 2003, 154; Scheel-Ybert et al. 2003, 110). This interpretation has been based on the fact that systematic excavations of the Jabuticabeira II site (Santa Catarina state) revealed that many bivalve shells were closed, indicating they had not been consumed prior to accumulation (Klokler 2008, 244). It is also clear that shells played an important role during funerary rituals: in the same site, heaps of shells covered both the individual hyperflexed burials and the group burials (Gaspar et al. 2008, 326; Klokler 2008, 123).

Fish: a Main Course for the Living and a Gift for the Dead

Once it was established that the shellmound-builders' diet focused on fish, which are found in almost all layers, zooarchaeologists tried to determine which species were being caught. In the case of Jabuticabeira II, species distribution is largely constant across time and space (Klokler 2001, 108). Zooarchaeological and isotopic studies have provided no evidence for seasonality (De Masi 2001, 112; Klokler 2001, 134). Overall, it seems the daily menu was limited to just a few species all the year round. For instance at Jabuticabeira II, 84 per cent of the fish assemblage consisted of three main species – *Micropogonias furnieri* (47 per cent of MNI), *Ariidae* (about 27 per cent) and *Archosargus probatocephalus* (about 10 per cent) – all of which are found in lake environments (Klokler 2001, 107). The abundant presence of *Mugil* sp. in certain stratigraphic layers, and the fact that this taxon lives in shoals, suggest the use of fishing nets or similar implements (Klokler 2001, 109).

Fish were so important to shellmound dwellers that they not only based their diet on them but offered fish to their deceased. Big fish appear to have been given as grave-goods whilst little ones seem to have been preferred as a feast food for the mourners. For example, one of the burials at Jabuticabeira II contained 55 fish (interpreted as offering), 46 fish recovered from the hearth on the top of burials (seen as food for the feast) while a further 395 fish were found in the sediment used to cover the hearth after the funerary ritual (Klokler 2001, 110).

The symbolic importance of fish is also clear from the material culture. Sites in southern Brazil have produced around 250 beautiful polished figurines representing fish (Fig. 1b) although, admittedly, other animals are also depicted. Almost all of the figurines have a dish-shaped cavity, interpreted as having held special substances used during rituals (Prous 1991, 233).

Stable Isotope Studies: You Are What You Eat

So far, stable isotope studies of shellmound skeletons have focused mainly on sites in Santa Catarina. The subsistence of those groups can be characterized, perhaps unsurprisingly, as a marine diet, indicated by high values of nitrogen (around 14‰) and carbon (around -13‰) (De Masi 2001, 112). At some sites, like Jabuticabeira II, values are even higher (carbon: -10.01–-11.90‰; nitrogen: 16.39–22.9‰ – Richards et al. 2007, 17–18; Klokler, 2008, 274, 307). Apparently there is no difference in fish intake between individuals exhumed from more recent sites or layers with and without pottery in Santa Catarina state. In all cases diet is clearly marine-based, although some groups have manifested some variation. For instance, analysis of the human remains from the site of Morro do Ouro returned isotopic values suggestive of a more terrestrial diet (carbon around -12‰ and nitrogen 10‰), probably indicating higher consumption of plants, possibly maize (De Masi 2001, 112). This is interesting given that analysis of the human remains from this site indicated a fairly high frequency of dental caries, indicative of a carbohydrate-rich diet (Turner II 1979, 631; Larsen 1997, 67 – see below).

The presence of some individuals with a more terrestrial diet, as well as the rich flora of the surrounding environment, indicate that plant consumption cannot be ignored when studying the subsistence patterns of those groups.

Palaeobotany

The importance of plant-use to shellmound dwellers is still not fully understood: the macroscopic plant remains have provided little evidence other than burnt coconuts, seeds and stone tools associated with plant processing (Kneip 1994, 4; Lima 1999–2000, 280). The presence of pottery fragments on the top of the upper layers of some of these sites has been considered as evidence of incipient agriculture or plant management (Beck

1972, 73). However, the skeletons from Santa Catarina found in the pottery-associated layers had a lower frequency of dental caries (Wesolowski 2000, 123) than that expected for agricultural groups – Turner II (1979, 625) has suggested 2.3 to 26.9 per cent – making it unlikely that the presence of pottery was related to plant domestication.

For subsistence reconstruction, settlement patterns are of utmost importance. Most of the shellmounds are located in the vicinity of sandy beach ridges covered by the 'restinga' ecosystem (a mosaic of different vegetation types that spreads inland from the shore on most of the Brazilian coastal plain). Its plant communities vary from sparse and open types, with herbaceous and scrub formations, to dense evergreen forests, extremely rich in plant foods (Scheel-Ybert et al. 2003, 126). Recently, anthracological studies have indicated that the shellmound dwellers were indeed exploiting the restinga ecosystem, utilizing a great diversity of seeds, fruits and tuberous plants such as *Dioscorea, Gramineae, Cyperaceae*, and *Typha domingensis* (Scheel-Ybert et al. 2003, 119). The study of plant microfossils such as phytoliths, pollen and starch grains have also provided evidence to suggest that plant-use was more significant that originally understood (Reinhard et al. 2001, 115; Boyadjian 2007, 133; Boyadjian et al. 2007, 1623; Wesolowski 2007, 149).

When plants are chewed, be it for feeding, medicinal purposes or artefact production, they may leave fragments which are later incorporated in the matrix of dental calculus (Reinhard et al. 2001, 112). Although the taxonomic identification of plants through the analysis of starch grains and phytoliths is not simple, it is sometimes possible to make reasonable taxa identification (Piperno and Holst 1998, 766; Piperno 2006, 27). Studies of plant microfossils preserved in dental calculus from inhumations at coastal sites in Santa Catarina show a positive correlation between greater frequencies of carious lesions and higher concentrations of starch grains present in dental calculus. Conversely sites where the human population exhibit low frequencies of dental caries (e.g. 6 per cent at Jabuticabeira II) also show lower concentrations of starch grains (Boyadjian 2007, 121). The presence of starch grains and phytoliths point to an intake of tubers (including yam, sweet potato, *Araceae*), and possibly maize and products that originated from palm processing (Wesolowski 2007, 170). Differences observed in terms of the relative proportion of these plants in the studied sites suggest that ecological, temporal and perhaps cultural factors were playing a role in food choice (Wesolowski 2007, 171).

Besides providing valuable information about the types of plants ingested, starch from dental calculus can also inform us about cooking practices. For example, around 22 per cent of the starch grains from the Jabuticabeira II material presented morphological modifications, a feature attributed to cooking procedures (Boyadjian 2007, 51). The presence of diatoms corroborated the aquatic nature of the diet in Jabuticabeira II, whereas dark fragments suggest that ashes were consumed (accidentally or as a spice) with cooked or roasted food, or that they were used for medicinal purposes (Boyadjian 2007, 63).

Palaeopathology

Human remains exhumed from Brazilian coastal shellmounds have been studied for more than half a century and have provided important information about the behaviour and lifestyle of shellmound populations.

Dental Pathologies: Classic Pattern of Diseases Found in Coastal Groups

As is seen in other coastal groups, the Brazilian shellmound populations show high levels of dental wear and, generally, low frequencies of caries, calculus, abscesses and ante-mortem tooth loss (Mendonça de Souza 1995, 202; Okumura and Eggers 2005, 275; Scheel-Ybert et al. 2003, 120; Neves and Wesolowski 2002, 387; Wesolowski 2000, 138). Figure 6.2 shows that, with the exception of the sites of Morro do Ouro and Rio Comprido Lower, all the groups had less than a four per cent rate of dental caries, which is closer to the level (0.00–5.3 per cent) expected for hunter-gather populations than that for agriculturalists (Turner II, 1979, 625). The low rates of periodontal disease are perhaps surprising given the excessive dental wear observed for the population: dental wear can cause loss of contact between adjacent teeth and irritation of nearby soft tissues, followed by inflammation and subsequent infection (Ortner and Putschar 1981, 442). Recently, the high dental wear was attributed to the inadvertent chewing of abrasive substances, such as sand, phytoliths and fragments of shellfish and fish bones (Reinhard et al. 2001, 115; Littleton and Frohlich 1993, 443; Machiarelli 1989, 582).

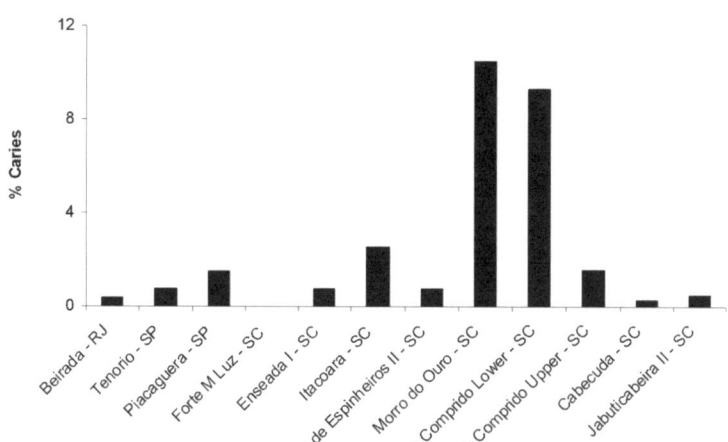

Figure 6.2. Percentage of teeth affected by caries per site (after Okumura and Eggers 2005, 269; Scheel-Ybert et al. 2003, 120). 'Rio Comprido Upper' and 'Rio Comprido Lower' refer to skeletons found in upper and lower layers of the same site.

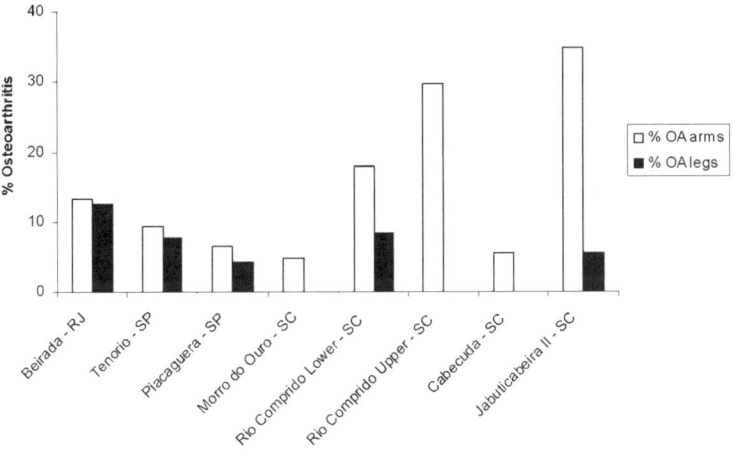

Figure 6.3. Percentage of osteoarthritis (OA) observed in arms and legs in different sites (after Okumura and Eggers 2005, 270; Petronilho 2003, 88). 'Rio Comprido Upper' and 'Rio Comprido Lower' refer to skeletons found in upper and lower layers of the same site.

Auditory Exostoses: Abnormal Bone Formation in Response to Aquatic Activity

Auditory exostoses are bone masses located in the external auditory canal. Because these bone formations were observed in coastal groups, and since water and atmospheric temperature as well as wind-effect play a pivotal role in the development of this trait, it was traditionally used as a proxy for aquatic activities (Kennedy 1986, 412). Nonetheless, it should be used cautiously in tropical and subtropical regions because it may fail to form despite aquatic activities, especially when water temperature is above 19°C, atmospheric temperature is high and the wind-chill is low (Okumura et al. 2007a, 564; 2007b, 471). However, frequencies of up to 50 per cent of individuals with auditory exostosis exhumed from southern shellmound sites (where environmental conditions are suitable for its development) support the idea that aquatic activities, mainly related to food acquisition, were being performed (Okumura et al. 2007a, 561; 2007b, 470).

Osteoarthritis: Wear and Tear Related to Fishing

Osteoarthritis, the loss of cartilage and subsequent bony lesions resulting from repetitive use of joints (Aufderheide and Rodriguez-Martin 1998, 93) is often used as a marker of activity intensity in prehistoric populations. Skeletal analysis of several shellmound sites (Fig. 6.3) show that, among adults, the upper limbs were significantly more affected by osteoarthritis than the lower ones (Rodrigues-Carvalho, 2004, 154; Okumura and Eggers 2005, 277; Neves 1986, 53; Scheel-Ybert et al. 2003, 120; Petronilho 2005, 128). The minimal stress-load observed in the lower limbs can be interpreted as indicating the short walking distances needed for resource procurement, which supports the idea resource abundance and predictability, as well as a fair degree of sedentarism. Activities like swimming, diving, rowing, throwing of fishing nets, and carrying baskets full of seafood could explain the upper limbs being more affected by osteoarthritis (Mendonça de Souza 1995, 231; Rodrigues-Carvalho, 2004, 188–189).

Conclusion

The integration of different fields of investigation, including zooarchaeology, stable isotopic analyses, palaeobotany and palaeopathology, allows a fairly good reconstruction of diet and lifestyle among the late Holocene coastal shellmound groups in Brazil. In the last two decades, many conventional ideas on shellmound lifestyle have been challenged through systematic studies that have provided a more complete and reliable picture. After centuries of speculation, we now know that the shellmound dwellers were not small mobile groups of hunter-gatherers who left behind mounds of food waste. On the contrary, there is now a growing evidence for sedentarism and greater social complexity.

Zooarchaeological and stable isotope analyses have shown that fish was remarkably important not just because the shellmound groups' diet was based on them but also because of their symbolic importance, evidenced by the recovery of stone figurines representing fish, as well as whole fish deposited as burial offerings. Indirect evidence for the importance of marine resources can be found in studies showing high incidence of auditory exostosis, a marker of aquatic activities, and a higher degree of osteoarthrosis in the upper than the lower limbs, which might be associated with the habit of swimming, diving, rowing, and throwing fishing nets. Although the macroscopic study of dental pathologies and stable isotope studies point to a diet usually poor in carbohydrates, the relative importance of plant consumption by these groups has been highlighted in the recent past thanks to studies focused on phytoliths, starch grains and anthracology.

Undoubtedly, further studies will help to clarify and enrich our understanding of the shellmound groups from southern Brazil.

Acknowledgements

Financial support was received from FAPESP. We would like to specially thank Naomi Sykes and Claire Newton for organizing the 3rd Conference on Food and Drink in Archaeology at the University of Nottingham. We would also like to thank all authors that kindly made data available to be included in this article.

References

Aufderheide, A.C. and Rodríguez-Martín, C. 1998. *The Cambridge Encyclopedia of Human Paleopathology* (Cambridge).

Beck, A. 1972. *A Variação do Conteúdo Cultural dos Sambaquis – Litoral de Santa Catarina*. PhD dissertation, University of São Paulo.

Boyadjian, C.H.C. 2007. *Análise do Calculo Dental em Sambaquieiros*. MPhil thesis, University of São Paulo.

——, Eggers, S and Reinhard, K.J. 2007. 'Dental wash: a problematic method for extracting microfossil from teeth', *Journal of Archaeological Science* 34, 1622–1628.

Chmyz, I. 1976. 'A ocupação do litoral dos estados do Paraná e Santa Catarina por povos ceramistas', *Estudos Brasileiros (Curitiba)* 1, 7–43.

De Masi, M.A.N. 2001. 'Pescadores coletores da costa sul do Brasil', *Pesquisas (série Antropologia)* 57, 1–136.

De Blasis, P.A.D., Fish, S.K., Gaspar, M.D. and Fish, P.R. 1998. 'Some references for the discussion of complexity among sambaqui moundbuilders from the Southern shores of Brazil', *Revista de Arqueologia Americana* 15, 75–105.

De Blasis, P., Kneip, A., Scheel–Ybert, R., Giannini, P.C. and Gaspar, M.D. 2007. 'Sambaquis e paisagem: dinâmica natural e arqueologia regional no litoral do sul do Brasil', *Arqueología Suramericana* 3, 28–61.

Figuti, L. 1993. 'O homem pré-histórico, o molusco e o sambaqui: considerações sobre a subsistência dos povos sambaquieiros', *Revista do Museu de Arqueologia e Etnologia (USP)* 3, 67–80.

Gaspar, M.D. 1998. 'Considerations of the sambaquis of the Brazilian coast', *Antiquity* 72, 592–615.

—— 2003. 'Aspectos da organização social de pescadores-coletores: região compreendida entre a ilha Grande e o delta do Paraíba do Sul', *Pesquisas (série Antropologia)* 59, 1–163.

——, De Blasis P., Fish S. K., and Fish P. R. 2008. 'Sambaqui (Shell Mound) Societies of Coastal Brazil', in Silverman, H., and Isbell, W. H. (eds) *Handbook of South American Archaeology* (New York), 319–335.

Kennedy, G.E. 1986. 'The relationship between exostoses and cold water: a latitudinal analysis', *American Journal of Physical Anthropololgy* 71, 401–415.

Klokler, D. 2001. *Construindo ou Deixando um Sambaqui? Análise de Sedimento de um Sambaqui do Litoral Meridional Brasileiro – Processos Formativos. Região de Laguna–SC*. MPhil thesis, University of São Paulo.

—— 2008. *Food for body and soul: mortuary ritual in shell mounds (Laguna, Brazil)*. PhD dissertation, University of Arizona.

Kneip, L.M. 1994. 'Cultura material e subsistência das populações pré-históricas de Saquarema, RJ', *Documento de Trabalho, Série Arqueologia N2 (Museu Nacional, Univ. Fed. Rio de Janeiro)* 2, 1–120.

Larsen, C.S. 1997. *Bioarchaeology: Interpreting Behavior from the Human Skeleton* (Cambridge).

Lima, T.A. 1999–2000. 'Em busca dos frutos do mar: os pescadores-coletores do litoral centro-sul do Brasil', *Revista USP* 44, 270–327.

Littleton, J. and Frohlich, B. 1993. 'Fish-eaters and farmers: dental pathology in the Arabian Gulf', *American Journal of Physical Anthropology* 92, 427–447.

Macchiarelli, R. 1989. 'Prehistoric "fish-eaters" along the eastern Arabian coasts: dental variation, morphology, and oral health in the Ra's al-Hamra community (Qurum, Sultanate of Oman, 5th–4th millennia BC)', *American Journal of Physical Anthropology* 78, 575–594.

Mendonça de Souza, S.M.F. 1995. *Estresse, Doença e Adaptabilidade: Estudo Comparativo de dois Grupos Pré-históricos em Perspectiva Biocultural*. PhD dissertation, ENSP/FIOCRUZ.

Neves, W.A. 1986. 'Incidência e distribuição de osteoartrites em grupos coletores do Litoral do Paraná: uma abordagem osteobiográfica', *Clio* 6, 47–62.

—— 1988. 'Paleogenética dos grupos pré-históricos do litoral sul do Brasil (Paraná e Santa Catarina)', *Pesquisas Antropologia* 43.

—— and Wesolowski, V. 2002. 'Economy, nutrition and disease in prehistoric coastal Brazil: a case study from the State of Santa Catarina', in Steckel, R.H. and Rose, J.C. (eds) *The Backbone of History: Health and Nutrition in the Western Hemisphere* (Cambridge), 376–402.

Okumura, M.M.M. 2008. 'Diversidade morfológica craniana, microevolução e ocupação pré-histórica da costa brasileira', *Pesquisas Antropologia* 66.

——. Accepted. 'Do cultural markers reflect biological affinities? A test using prehistoric ceramist and non-ceramist groups from coastal Brazil', in Roksandic M. (ed.) *Shellmounds*.

——, Boyadjian, C.H.C., Eggers, S. 2007a. 'Auditory exostoses as an aquatic activity marker: a comparison of coastal and inland skeletal remains from Tropical and Subtropical regions of Brazil', *American Journal of Physical Anthropology* 132, 558–567.

——, Boyadjian, C.H.C., Eggers, S. 2007b. 'An evaluation of auditory exostoses in 621 prehistoric skulls from coastal Brazil', *Ear, Throat and Nose Journal* 86(8), 468–472.

——, Eggers, S. 2005. 'The people from Jabuticabeira II: reconstruction of the way of life in a Brazilian shellmound', *Homo: Journal of Comparative Biology* 55, 263–281.

Ortner, D. and Putschar, W. 1981. *Identification of Pathological Conditions in Human Skeletal Remains* (Washington DC).

Petronilho, C. 2005. *Comprometimento articular como um marcador de atividades em um grande sambaqui-cemitério*. MSc thesis, University of São Paulo.

Piperno, D.R. 2006. *Phytoliths: A Comprehensive Guide for Archaeologists and Palaeoecologists* (Altamira Press).

—— and Holst, I. 1998. 'The presence of starch grains on Prehistoric stone tools from the humid Neotropics: indications of early tuber use and agriculture in Panama', *Journal of Archaeological Science* 25, 765–776

Prous, A. 1991. *Arqueologia Brasileira* (Brasília).

Reinhard, K.J., Mendonça de Souza, S.F., Rodrigues, C., Kimerle E. and Dorsey-Vinton, S. 2001. 'Microfossils in dental calculus: a new perspective on diet and dental disease', in Williams, E. (ed.) *Human Remains: Conservation, Retrieval and Analysis* (Oxford, BAR International Series 934), 113–118.

Richards, M., de Blasis, P. and Eggers, S. 2007. 'Stable isotopes and what they reveal about paleodiet in Jabuticabeira II', *Anais do XIV Congresso da Sociedade de Arqueologia Brasileira* (Florianópolis).

Rodrigues-Carvalho, C. 2004. *Marcadores de Estresse Ocupacional em Populações Sambaquieiras do Litoral fluminense*. PhD dissertation, Escola Nacional de Saúde Pública, Fiocruz, Rio de Janeiro.

Scheel-Ybert, R., Eggers, S., Wesolowski, V., Petronilho, C.C., Boyadjian, C.H., De Blasis, P.A.D., Barbosa-Buimarães, M. and Gaspar, M.D. 2003. 'Novas perspectivas na reconstituição do modo de vida dos sambaquieiros: uma abordagem multidisciplinar', *Revista Arqueologia (SAB)* 16, 109–137.

Turner II, C.G. 1979. 'Dental anthropological indications of agriculture among the Jomon people of Central Japan', *American Journal Physical Anthropology* 51, 619–635.

Wesolowski, V. 2000. *A Prática da Horticultura Entre Os Construtores de Shellmounds e Acampamentos Litorâneos da Região da Baía de São Francisco, Santa Catarina: Uma Abordagem Bio-antropológica*. MPhil thesis, University of São Paulo.

—— 2007. *Cáries, Desgaste, Cálculos Dentários e Micro-resíduos da Dieta Entre Grupos Pré-históricos do Litoral norte de Santa Catarina: é Possível Comer Amido e Não Ter Cárie?* PhD dissertation, University of São Paulo.

Between Sacrifice and Consumption: the Deceased as Metaphorical Food in Iron Age Veneto

Elisa Perego, University College, London

The aim of this paper is to explore whether the dead were conceived as metaphorical food in Iron Age Veneto (Italy). This hypothesis is based on the fact that Venetic funerary practices persistently adopted culinary and banqueting vessels as urns and tomb-containers. Similar practices are noted for other archaeological cultures that, together with the anthropological literature, emphasize how metaphorical ties between the deceased and food are often created in mortuary rituals worldwide. In this work I discuss whether Venetic individuals were compared to specific foodstuffs according to their sex, age and rank on the basis of the typology of the culinary vessels adopted as urns.

The Dead as Food in Anthropology and Archaeology

Anthropological research has long recognized that, across cultures, there are strong ties between food consumption and death, often elaborated in funerary rituals. Cannibalism, for example, either practised in reality or alluded to through symbolism and mythology, clearly entails the conceptualization of the dead as edible flesh (Bloch 1985; Conklin 2001; Oestigaard 2004; Young 1989; Parry 1982; Strathern 1982; Viveiros de Castro 1992). Funerals in northern India involve the symbolic consumption of the deceased, who is literally represented as food (Parry 1985). A metaphorical parallel is drawn between the physical process of digestion, through which the body eliminates the waste products of food and refines the nourishment, and the mortuary ritual, which requires the elimination of the dead individual's sins and the refinement of his/her own pure essence. Among the Berawan of Borneo, it has been suggested that a metaphorical connection is created between fermentation and putrefaction (Huntington and Metcalf 1979, 56–57). The same types of jars are used both for the production of rice wine and the temporary storage of the decaying corpse. The identical, albeit reversed, process is adopted to produce both wine and ancestors. The fermentation of rice produces the liquor and entails the removal of the useless solid rice skin, whereas the putrefaction of the body produces the bones of the ancestors and involves the elimination of the useless liquids of decay. The Yanomami of Venezuela actually consume the burnt bones of their dead which are ground in a mortar and then mixed into a soup drunk by the community (Lizot 1985).

Similar ties between death and eating have been recognized in past contexts (e.g. Hamilakis 1998), especially in the case of cremation, which may entail the symbolic cooking of human flesh (Oestigaard 2000). In Iron Age Etruria, the burial of cremated individuals in vessels originally used as liquid-containers – such as biconical urns, *amphorae*, laminated bronze short-necked vessels and clay *krater*-urns – probably implied the elaboration of symbolic ties between the dead and food (Riva 2010). This metaphorical correspondence is even clearer during the *Orientalizing* period (*ca.* seventh century BC) with the deposition of cremated élite males in wine-containers (impasto *olle*) and bronze cauldrons used for meat-boiling: a clear reference to the ritual banquet, whose essential components were alcohol and meat. It is important to recognize that these cremation practices were taking place at a time when inhumation was the norm. This would have highlighted the exceptional nature of the individuals and their incineration may have been conceived as a sacrificial act in which the warrior was symbolically compared to the animal victims cooked in the cauldron (Riva 2010). Similar ritual practices entailing the creation of symbolic links between the dead and food may have been also elaborated in Iron Age Veneto, as I discuss in the following paragraphs.

The Mortuary Domain in Iron Age Veneto

The Veneti, a population of probable Indo-European origin, created a complex and hierarchical society in north-east Italy during the first millennium BC (Fig. 7.1). Knowledge of local funerary rituals is mainly drawn from the cemeteries excavated at important settlements such as Este, Padua, Altino, Montebelluna, Oppeano and Gazzo Vr. (e.g. Capuis 2009; Capuis and Chieco Bianchi 1992; De Min et al. 2005; Manessi and Nascimbene 2003; Salzani 2001; *Veneti Antichi* 2008). At these sites, cremation was the most common ritual adopted but inhumation was practised as well. In the case of cremation, burnt human remains were separated from pyre debris and deposited in ceramic or metal vessels. Ceramic urns were occasionally placed in bucket-shaped bronze vessels (*situlae*) before their interment. Grave-goods – ornaments, tools, weapons and vessels with the meal for the dead – were also placed in the grave. When the tomb was closed, pyre debris was scattered over it and a small tumulus was erected. However, the structure of cremation graves could vary (Fig. 7.2). The most common tomb structure at the main settlement of Este was the so-called *cassetta*, a rectangular box of stone slabs. Less frequently urns were placed in wooden containers and large ceramic vessels (*dolia*), or directly in the soil without any protection (pit graves). More common at other sites such as Padua and Altino was the use of timber boxes and *dolia* as tomb-containers. Common to many Venetic cemeteries was the practice of reopening a grave to deposit more individuals, whose remains were sometimes mingled with the bones of the dead already buried in the tomb. On such occasions, part of the old dining set was intentionally scattered over the grave, possibly to provide room for the vessels belonging to the new dead (Vanzetti 1992).

Venetic tombs tended to coalesce into common burial mounds. Between the sixth and the fifth centuries BC some of the largest tumuli demonstrate a hierarchical arrangement in the graves' disposition, especially at Este and Padua: inhumations,

Between Sacrifice and Consumption

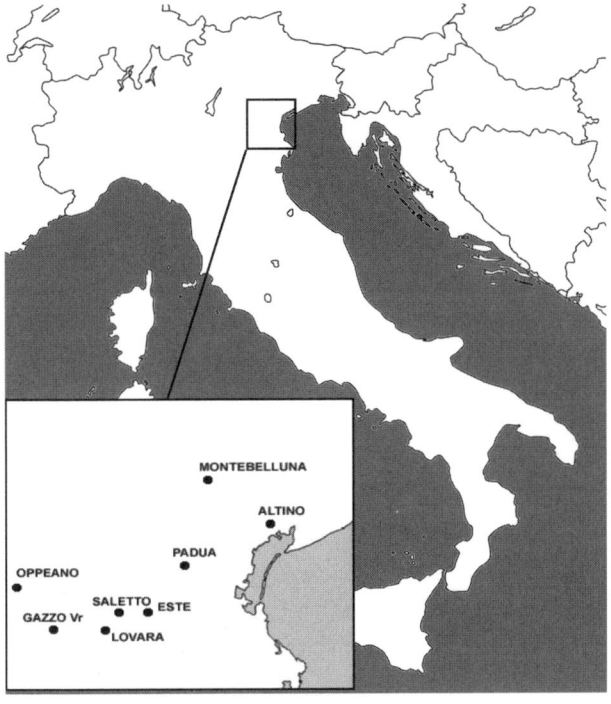

Figure 7.1. Map of Veneto with sites mentioned in the chapter (drawn by the author).

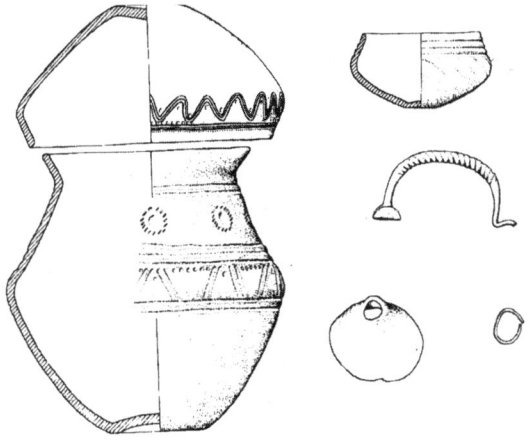

Figure 7.2. Grave assemblage from infant Gazzo Vr. Colombara tomb 34 (900–850 BC): biconical vessel used as urn; large bowl used as a lid; small bowl; arched fibula; ring and pierced shell valve (modified by the author after Salzani 2001).

small *cassette* and simple pit graves were arranged along the tumulus edge, in clearly subordinate positions, while cremated individuals accompanied by a wealth of grave-goods were placed in grand multiple tombs in the middle (Balista and Ruta Serafini 1992; Gambacurta et al. 2006).

In many cases, a dining or banqueting set, including an array of bronze and ceramic implements for food preparation and consumption, was placed at the bottom of the grave (Chieco Bianchi and Calzavara Capuis 1985; 2006; Perego 2010). Meals for the dead were arranged in bowls, high-footed cups and 'plates' which sometimes have been found to contain the residues of solid foodstuffs (e.g. Chieco Bianchi and Calzavara Capuis 1985, 272). Larger vessels such as *situlae* and *situliformi* were possibly employed as the Venetic equivalent of Greek '*kraters*', namely as liquid-containers in which alcoholic and/or other prestigious beverages were mixed with water and other substances before redistribution. High-handled cups (*tazze ad ansa soprelevata*), ladles and, later, jugs were used to remove the beverage from the '*krater*' and to pour it. Strainers were probably used to filter alcohol.

Drinking vessels included *bicchieri* of local production (similar in form to modern glasses) and imported Greek cups such as *skyphoi* and *kylikes*. The preparation and consumption of solid foods was alluded to by the deposition of slices, roasting spits and possibly knives and axes. Rarely, however, was the entire assemblage such as I have described above buried in a single grave. Differences in the composition of the service were probably due to the social standing of the deceased; wealthy tombs were generally endowed with more luxurious banqueting sets than simple graves. It seems possible that other factors, such as sex and age, also influenced choices about the type of vessels deposited in funerary contexts. Similar criteria, namely the age, gender and rank of the deceased, may have also determined what kind of vessel shape was used as an urn. In order to determine whether this was the case, I examined funerary data from six Venetic localities: Este, Saletto and Padua in central Veneto, Montebelluna in the Piave River valley, Altino on the Adriatic Sea and Lovara in the Verona countryside.

Data and Methods

The dataset considered in this paper includes 366 cases (i.e. burial urns) but the geographic distribution of this evidence is not uniform. The vast majority of the cases analysed (319 urns, 88 per cent) are from Este, with finds from the cemeteries of Benvenuti, Ricovero, Alfonsi and Capodaglio. Twenty urns (5.5 per cent) have been recovered from Padua and 19 from Montebelluna (5.2 per cent). Only eight urns in total (2.2 per cent) are from Altino, Lovara and Saletto, whose cemeteries still await examination in published form. The chronological span of the evidence ranges between the ninth and the second centuries BC, with a peak in the sixth century (26.3 per cent of the total). Where osteological analysis of the cremated remains is available (Drusini et al. 1998; Drusini et al. 2006; Onisto 2003; Ovidi 2006; Salzani et al. 2000), the sex and the age of the deceased have been correlated to the types of the vessels adopted as

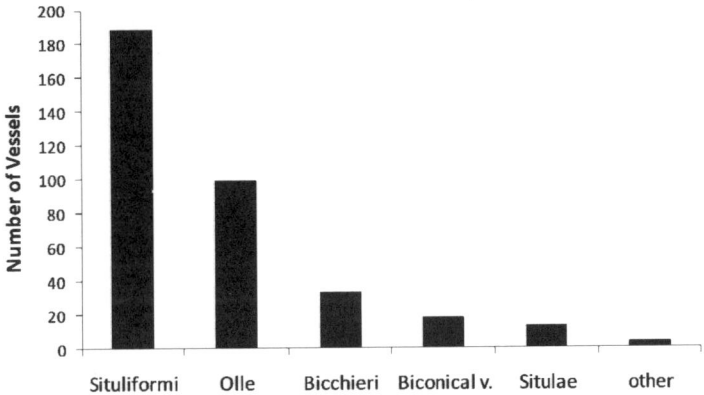

Figure 7.3. Total number of urns attested per class of vessels (drawn by the author).

urns, as I attempt to detect the criteria which may have determined the adoption of a specific container in relation to the status of the deceased. The gender of the dead has been established in the case of 95 ossuaries (25.7 per cent), the age in the case of 169 (46 per cent). Occasional errors in the osteological analysis presented must be expected as the analysis of cremated remains is notoriously difficult.

The identification of specific containers as culinary vessels has been based on iconographic and archaeological evidence, including the presence of solid food residues in a range of ceramics placed in the tomb (Chieco Bianchi and Calzavara Capuis 1985; 2006). Chemical analysis of charred remains and food encrustations is rarely carried out in Venetic archaeology. This lack of documentation is regrettable, particularly for those vessels which must have contained liquids, as in this case it is impossible to identify the kinds of beverages buried in the grave. Statistical analysis (undertaken using SPSS) of the composition of funerary dining sets is based on a sample of 89 graves from the Este Benvenuti cemetery (Chieco Bianchi and Calzavara Capuis 2006). The sample includes only those vessels intentionally placed in the tomb-container. The fragmented ceramics often recovered from the grave mound and filling are not considered in this analysis since it is sometimes difficult to demonstrate their association with the tomb.

Results

Statistical analysis (undertaken using SPSS) shows that in my database ceramic bucket-shaped vessels (*situliformi*) are by far the most common containers adopted as urns (189 occurrences, 51.6 per cent) (Fig. 7.3). However, *situliformi* declined in popularity in the late Iron Age and went out of use in the third century BC. *Olle* are also a common vessel shape in my sample, being utilized as urns in 99 cases (27 per cent). *Bicchieri* and *vasi a bicchere* were used as urns more rarely (33 occurrences, 9 per cent). Biconical vessels were employed as cinerary urns until the seventh century BC (14 cases, 3.8 per cent), when they went out of use. *Situlae* were adopted as urns from the eighth to the third centuries BC: always in wealthy graves (13 cases, 3.6 per cent). Slightly more widespread – albeit still rare – was the employment of *situlae* as containers of ceramic urns. Other types of vessels, including *dolia* (large ceramic foodstuff containers), small jars, jugs and cups, were employed very rarely as urns (3 per cent in total). On the basis of preliminary statistical analysis, no significant relation has been detected between the adoption of a particular vessel-type and the gender of the deceased. It must be emphasized, however, that the criteria for selection of any one vessel may have revolved around specific characteristics of the vessel (e.g. decoration) which are not taken into account in my analysis. The deposition of more than one individual in approximately 20 per cent of the urns further complicates this analysis, as well as the existence of possible depositional variations related to the burials' chronology and location. In particular, the results of my analysis may have been influenced by the absolute predominance of material from Este in the sample. Clearer is the association of children with *bicchieri* and small *olle*, although infants were also buried in other containers. The reason for this preference is probably motivated by the vessels' smaller dimensions. However, the possibility that these pots were selected as infant urns for specifically ritual reasons cannot be discounted. Bronze *situlae* were employed as funerary vessels only in the case of élite or very wealthy depositions, regardless of the gender and age of the deceased (Chieco Bianchi and Calzavara Capuis 1985; 2006).

Culinary Vessels as Urns in Iron Age Veneto

The aim of this section is to discuss the similarity between urns and culinary vessels and to establish their precise pre-funerary function. As I elaborate below, the types of vessels used as funerary urns in Veneto generally have parallels in similar examples either placed at the bottom of the grave as part of the funerary dining set or used in everyday and ritual food storage, preparation and consumption in local settlements and sanctuaries. The similarity between funerary urns and culinary vessels in dimension, shape and decoration is sometimes striking (e.g. Chieco Bianchi and Calzavara Capuis 2006: 223, 355), emphasizing the ritual interchangeability between the two. Even when specific types of urns were produced expressly for the grave, their shape and/or decoration were often reminiscent of vessels commonly used as food or liquid containers. The latter consideration is of a paramount importance for my hypothesis. The fact that the Veneti adopted culinary vessels and liquid containers (or their copies) as urns, even when they could have produced completely different shapes, suggests that their choice was meaningful and deliberate. It is also important to emphasize that urns need not be imitations of culinary vessels. Although food containers, due to their shapes and dimensions, are often an obvious choice for the deposition of cremated human remains, other options are well documented in the funerary record. For example, hut-shaped cinerary urns (*urne a capanna*) became common in some Italian areas between the late Bronze Age and the early Iron Age (Bietti Sestrieri and De Santis 2006: 81).

The metaphorical connection between food preparation and consumption and the funerary sphere in Veneto may have been also reinforced by the widespread use of bowls and cups as urn-lids, although this aspect of the Venetic mortuary ritual is not discussed here. Further, it is occasionally possible to demonstrate that a specific urn had been used directly for food preparation before interment. This might have been the case of the large bronze *situlae* employed as urn-containers in the élite Ricovero tomb 232 (sixth century BC), whose external surface shows clear evidence of exposure to fire (Chieco Bianchi and Calzavara Capuis 1985, 273). The evidence of pre-funerary wear and repair found on other *situlae*-urns further suggests these vessels may actually have been used before burial. The intentional removal of the handles from some *situlae* and other vessel-shapes at the time of the funeral also indicates these containers were initially made for real use or to resemble real vessels (e.g. Chieco Bianchi and Calzavara Capuis 2006, 281).

Also significant may be the widespread employment of coarse domestic *situliformi* as urns throughout the eighth century BC, even in wealthy graves where more luxurious tableware, prepared specifically for the grave, was included in the dining service (Chieco Bianchi and Calzavara Capuis 1985, 46). The careful selection of these culinary vessels of everyday use must have been motivated by specific ritual needs and possibly implied a deliberate reference to food preparation. The evidence of pre-funerary repair found on the *situliforme*-ossuary from Ricovero tomb 133 further indicates that these pots were actually used before their deposition in the grave (ibid., 49). The employment of domestic vessels as urns continued into later periods, especially in the case of infant depositions and simple pit graves (ibid., 220). However, this practice can also be recognized in more prestigious burials (e.g. ibid., 263).

The employment of large *situliformi* (average height 20–25cm) as '*kraters*' at the funerary banquet is suggested by the occasional deposition of high-handled cups inside them (e.g. Bagolan 1998, 120). This hypothesis is strengthened by the *situliformi*'s shape itself, clearly reminiscent of that of bronze *situlae*, whose adoption as liquid-containers is demonstrated by both archaeological evidence and iconography (see below). Furthermore, the surface of *situliformi* placed in wealthy graves was occasionally burnished or adorned with metallic studs to reproduce the metallic shine of *situlae* and enhance the similarity between the two; *situlae*, in turn, were sometimes shaped and decorated to resemble *situliformi* (Capuis and Chieco Bianchi 1992). Smaller *situliformi* (average height 12–15cm), placed at the bottom of the grave, were presumably adopted as liquid or food containers but probably not as real *kraters*, unless they represented miniature versions of the larger examples. *Situliformi* were included in the dining service of only 18 per cent of the 98 Benvenuti graves analysed in this paper, whereas *olle* appeared in 44 per cent of tombs from the same cemetery. The reason for the disproportion between the widespread use of *situliformi* as urns and their relatively rare inclusion in the funerary banqueting set is unclear.

The adoption of *olle* as culinary vessels is testified by their widespread diffusion in settlement sites (e.g. De Min et al. 2005; Malnati et al. 1996). Large domestic *olle* were sporadically employed as tomb-containers (Chieco Bianchi and Calzavara Capuis 1985, 118–119). The *olle* included in funerary dining sets were generally smaller than those used as urns (average height 8–15cm vs. 20cm) and must have contained reduced portions of liquid or food. The smallest examples (*ollette bicchiere*) were possibly used as drinking vessels as well as infant urns. Larger *olle* bearing greater resemblance to those employed as urns were occasionally placed in graves as part of the funerary banqueting set (e.g. Chieco Bianchi and Calzavara Capuis 2006, 241; Paiola 1998, 192). The deposition of a high-handled cup in a small *olla* from a multiple grave from Este, Ricovero tomb 21 (Paiola 1998, 191), would suggest that the vessel was used as a liquid-container, although its employment as a *krater* is improbable due to it being so small. The sporadic interment of *olle*, *bicchieri* and *situliformi* with lids may suggest that these vessels contained different foods vis-à-vis those buried without a cover: Chieco Bianchi and Calzavara Capuis (2006, 211) have argued that the lids may have been intended to prevent the evaporation of liquid placed inside.

Biconical vessels were generally not included in the funerary dining service (an exception is Ricovero tomb 177, Chieco Bianchi and Calzavara Capuis 1985, 150–152) and certain types seem to have been exclusively adopted as urns (Vanzetti 1992). The presence of biconical vessels in domestic contexts, however, demonstrates their employment for food preparation or storage (Chieco Bianchi and Calzavara Capuis 1985, 81–82). The use of *bicchieri* as drinking vessels was widespread at the Venetic funerary banquet. At Este Benvenuti, *bicchieri* were included in the dining set of 50 graves out of 89 (56.2 per cent). The average height of the *bicchieri* used for drinking purposes was around 12cm. *Bicchieri* of this size were employed as urns for small children (e.g. Chieco Bianchi and Calzavara Capuis 2006, 355). Larger examples (*vasi a bicchiere*) were used both as urns and culinary vessels or liquid-containers. For example, those *vasi a bicchieri* placed at the bottom of graves occasionally contained a high-handled cup (e.g. Chieco Bianchi and Calzavara Capuis 2006, 148), suggesting that they were used as *kraters*. The deposition of food remains in a few *bicchieri* from Este (Chieco Bianchi and Calzavara Capuis 2006, 183–184, 232) would indicate that these vessels were also used to contain solid food. The sporadic adoption of culinary and banqueting vessels, including *bicchieri*, *situlae* and *situliformi*, as containers of non-food funerary offerings (e.g. Chieco Chieco Bianchi and Calzavara Capuis 1985, 72; 2006, 154, 179, 186, 211, 215, 273) confirms a certain variability in the use of these shapes.

Other vessels such as *dolia*, cups, jugs, small jars (*orcioli*) and *situlae* were much less commonly employed as urns. More frequent was the adoption of *dolia* as tomb-containers, especially at Padua and Altino. *Dolia* were generally not included in funerary dining sets, but their employment as food containers is demonstrated by their widespread occurrence in settlement contexts (e.g. De Min et al. 2005; Malnati et al. 1996). Jugs similar to those used as urns in multiple Benvenuti tomb 230 (for a male) and Capodaglio tomb 4/1982 were often placed at the bottom of late Iron Age graves as part of the funerary drinking set (Chieco Bianchi and Calzavara Capuis 2006,

290). Jugs have also been recovered from several settlement sites and are represented on bronze laminas and figurines from the Baratella sanctuary at Este, where they are associated with female figures about to pour a liquid. The diffusion of jugs in Veneto, especially from the third century BC, was related to the adoption of new sympotic practices which implied a diverse way of serving the beverage, previously removed from the *krater* through ladles and high-handled cups (Chieco Bianchi and Calzavara Capuis 2006, 293). The small jar (*orciolo*) used as an urn in the (female) Ricovero tomb 128 (late ninth century) is similar to several *orcioli* unearthed in contemporary settlement contexts (Chieco Bianchi and Calzavara Capuis 1985, 41–42). Other *orcioli* probably employed as liquid-containers were placed in a few graves dated to the early Iron Age (Chieco Bianchi and Calzavara Capuis 1985; 2006).

The employment of bronze *situlae* as liquid-containers is testified by several ceremonial and élite drinking scenes embossed and engraved on bronze plaques found between the Po Valley and the Danube plain (e.g. Chieco Bianchi and Calzavara Capuis 2006, 321). The link between the *situlae* and drinking is also emphasized by the deposition of a complete bronze banqueting set including a *situla*, a *cista*, three strainers and a high-handled cup in one of the urns – a bronze *situla* itself – of the eighth-century BC élite Ricovero tomb 236 (Chieco Bianchi and Calzavara Capuis 1985; Iaia 2006). The association between the *situlae* and the strainers in Ricovero tomb 236, as well as the deposition of bronze *situlae* in exceptional graves, testify to the adoption of *situlae* as '*kraters*' at the Venetic aristocratic banquet, which probably entailed the consumption of alcohol. The burial of *situlae* exposed to fire before interment suggests that these vessels may have been also used for cooking, an instance documented elsewhere in late prehistoric Italy (e.g. Coen 2008, 163). Therefore, I would not exclude that Venetic *situlae* may have been employed for meat-boiling, like the Etruscan cauldrons, or for the preparation of other luxurious foods consumed at an élite banquet. The exceptional dimensions of the burnt *situlae* from Ricovero tomb 232 (height 40–50cm) clearly indicate the preparation of large amounts of food probably redistributed between the banqueters. The same ritual logic governed similar practices of hierarchical commensality in pre-Roman Italy, especially in the case of wine consumption, with the aristocrat taking control of food preparation and distribution (Iaia 2006; Riva 2010). The evidence discussed in this paper would suggest that the ideology of the sacrificial banquet spread into the Veneto, as well as into Etruria, and influenced Venetic choice in terms of ritual and symbolic expressions of the dynamics of power vis-à-vis subordination (Perego 2010).

Conclusion

In this paper I have discussed how the adoption of culinary vessels as urns and tomb-containers in Iron Age Veneto suggests that there were possibly deep metaphorical ties between local practices of food consumption and the funerary treatment of the deceased. Although it is impossible to demonstrate beyond doubt that the dead were conceived as metaphorical food, the evidence presented testifies that culinary vessels were at least considered appropriate recipients for human remains. The vessels employed as urns and tombs included liquid-containers (*situliformi*, *orcioli* and jugs), drinking vessels (*bicchieri* and *ollette bicchiere*) and foodstuff containers (large domestic *olle* and *dolia*). The scarcity of samples and the difficulty of establishing the precise pre-funerary function of the vessels adopted as urns undermines any attempt to identify a clear link between specific foods and the sex and age of the deceased. Noteworthy however is the adoption of bronze *situlae* as urns and urn-containers in élite depositions, with the possible elaboration of symbolic ties between the élite dead and ritual practices of food consumption, including the sacrificial banquet.

Acknowledgements

I want to thank Dr Naomi Sykes for her work and the anonymous referee for the useful comments which helped me to improve my paper. Many thanks to Dr Corinna Riva who allowed me to read her book when it was still unpublished.

References

Bagolan, M. 1998. 'Tomba 44', in Bianchin Citton, E., Gambacurta G. and Ruta Serafin, A. (eds.) in ....*Presso l'Adige Ridente....Recenti Rinvenimenti Archeologici da Este a Montagnana* (Padova), 117–129.

Balista, C. and Ruta Serafini, A. 1992. 'Este preromana. Nuovi dati sulle necropoli', in G. Tosi (ed.) *Este Antica dalla Preistoria all'Età Romana* (Este), 109–123.

Bietti Sestrieri, A. M. and De Santis, A. 2006. 'Il rituale funerario nel Lazio tra Età del Bronzo finale e prima Età del Ferro', in Von Eles, P. (ed.) *La Ritualità Funeraria tra Età del Ferro e Orientalizzante in Italia. Atti del Convegno. Verrucchio 26–27 Giugno 2002* (Pisa), 79–91.

Bloch, M. 1985. 'Almost eating the ancestors', *Man* 20(4), 631–646.

Capuis, L. 2009. *I Veneti. Civiltà e Cultura di un Popolo dell'Italia Preromana* (Milano).

—— and Chieco Bianchi, A.M. 1992. 'Este preromana. Vita e cultura', in G. Tosi (ed.) *Este Antica dalla Preistoria all'Età Romana* (Este), 41–108.

Chieco Bianchi, A. M. and Calzavara Capuis, L. 1985. *Le Necropoli di Casa di Ricovero, Casa Muletti Prosdocimi, Casa Alfonsi* (Roma).

—— and Calzavara Capuis, L. 2006. *La Necropoli di Villa Benvenuti* (Roma).

Coen, A. 2008. 'Il banchetto aristocratico e il ruolo della donna', in Silvestrini, M. and Sabbatini, T. (eds) *Potere e Splendore. Gli Antich Piceni a Matelica* (Rome), 159–165.

Conklin, B. A. 2001. *Consuming Grief: Compassionate Cannibalism in an Amazonian Society* (Austin).

De Min, M., Gambacurta, G. and Ruta Serafini, A. 2005. *La Città Invisibile. Padova Preromana: Trent'Anni di Scavi e Ricerche* (Bologna).

Drusini, A., Onisto, N. and Ranzato, C. 1998. 'Studio antropologico degli incinerati', in Bianchin Citton, E., Gambacurta, G. and Ruta Serafini, A. (eds) *Presso l'Adige Ridente....Recenti Rivenimenti Archeologici da Este a Montagnana* (Padova), 36–47.

Drusini, A. G., Carrara, N. and Onisto, N. 2006. 'Analisi dei resti ossei cremati', in Chieco Bianchi, A. M. and Calzavara Capuis, L. (eds) *La Necropoli di Villa Benvenuti* (Roma), 397–449.

Gambacurta, G., Locatelli, D., Marinetti, A. and Ruta Serafini, A. 2006. 'Delimitazione dello spazio e rituale funerario nel Veneto preromano', in Cresci Marrone, G. and Tirelli, M. (eds) *'Terminavit Sepulcrum'. I Recenti Funerari nelle Necropoli di Altino* (Roma), 9–40.

Hamilakis, Y. 1998. 'Eating the dead: mortuary feasting and the political economy of the memory in the Bronze Age Aegean', in Branigan, K. (ed.) *Cemetery and Society in the Aegean Bronze Age* (Sheffield), 115–132.

Huntington, R. and Metcalf, P. 1979. *Celebrations of Death: The Anthropology of Mortuary Ritual* (Cambridge).

Iaia, C. 2006. 'Servizi cerimoniali da Simposio in Bronzo del Primo Ferro in Italia Centro-Settentrionale', in Von Eles, P. (ed.) *La Ritualità Funeraria tra Età del Ferro e Orientalizzante in Italia. Atti del Convegno. Verrucchio 26–27 Giugno 2002* (Pisa), 103–110.

Lizot, J. 1985. *Tales of the Yanomami: Daily Life in the Venezuelan Forest* (Cambridge).

Malnati, L., Croce Da Villa, P. and Di Filippo Balestrazzi, E. 1996. *La Protostoria tra Sile e Tagliamento. Antiche Genti tra Veneto e Friuli* (Padova).

Manessi, P. and Nascimbene, A. 2003. *Montebelluna. Sepolture Preromane dalle Necropoli di S. Maria del Colle e Posmon* (Montebelluna).

Oestigaard, T. 2000. 'Sacrifices of raw, cooked and burnt humans', *Norwegian Archaeological Review* 33(1), 41–58.

—— 2004. 'Kings and cremation: royal funerals and sacrifices in Nepal', in Insoll, T. (ed.) *Belief in the Past. The Proceedings of the Manchester Conference on Archaeology and Religion* (Oxford, BAR International Series 1212), 115–124.

Onisto, N. 2003. 'Studio antropologico dei resti ossei cremati dalle necropoli di S. Maria del Colle e Posmon', in Manessi, P. and Nascimbene, A. (eds) *Montebelluna. Sepolture Preromane dalle Necropoli di S. Maria del Colle e Posmon* (Montebelluna), 299–313.

Ovidi, L. 2006. 'Necropoli casa di Ricovero: analisi antropologica e archeologica a confronto', in Chieco Bianchi, A. M. and Calzavara Capuis, L. (eds) *La Necropoli di Villa Benvenuti* (Roma), 477–484.

Paiola, S. 1998. 'Tomba 21', in Bianchin Citton, E., Gambacurta, G. and Ruta Serafini, A. (eds) *Presso l'Adige Ridente....Recenti Rivenimenti Archeologici da Este a Montagnana* (Padova), 180–194.

Parry, J. 1982. 'Sacrificial death and the necrophagous ascetic', in Bloch, M. and Parry, J. (eds) *Death and the Regeneration of Life* (Cambridge), 74–110.

—— 1985. 'Death and digestion: the symbolism of food and eating in North Indian mortuary rites', *Man* 20(4), 612–630.

Perego, E. 2010. 'Osservazioni Preliminari sul Banchetto Funerario Rituale nel Veneto Preromano: Acquisizione, Innovazione e Resistenza Culturale', in C. Mata Parreno, G. Pérez Jordà and J. Vives–Ferrandiz Sanchez (eds) *De la Cuina a la Taula. IV Reunio d'Economia en el I Millenni a.C.* Saguntum. Papeles del Laboratorio de Arqueologia de Valencia, Extra 9, 287–294.

Riva, C. 2010. *The Culture of Urbanization in Etruria c. 800–600 BC* (Cambridge).

Salzani, L. 2001. 'Tombe protostoriche dalla necropoli della Colombara (Gazzo Veronese)', *Padusa* 37, 83–132.

Salzani, L., Drusini, A. and Malnati, L. 2000. 'Orfeo in Veneto. La tomba 13 della Necropoli di Lovara (Villa Bartolomea)', *Quaderni di Archeologia del Veneto* 16, 138–148.

Strathern, A. 1982. 'Witchcraft, greed, cannibalism and death: some related themes from the New Guinea Highlands' in Bloch, M. and Parry, J. (eds) *Death and the Regeneration of Life* (Cambridge), 111–133.

Vanzetti, A. 1992. 'Le sepolture a incinerazione a più deposizioni nella Protostoria dell'Italia Nord-Orientale', *Rivista di Scienze Preistoriche* 44(1–2), 115–209.

Veneti Antichi 2008. *I Veneti Antichi: Novita' e Aggiornamenti* (Sommacampagna).

Viveiros de Castro, E. 1992. *From the Enemy's Point of View. Humanity and Divinity in an Amazonian Society* (Chicago).

Young, M. 1989 '"Eating the dead": mortuary transactions in Bwaidoka, Goodenough Island', in Damon, F. and Wagner, R. (eds) *Death Rituals and Life in the Societies of the Kula Ring* (Dekalb), 179–198.

A Different Kettle of Fish:
Food Diversity in Mesolithic Scotland

Catriona Pickard and Clive Bonsall, University of Edinburgh

In the opening paragraph of *Scotland: Archaeology and Early History*, Ritchie and Ritchie (1991, 13) noted that the 'great variety of the natural habitats, the interplay of sea, mountain, river and forest, provided many different environments for the hunting-gathering-fishing communities who made their way into Scotland from the south from about 7000 BC'. Although the timing and origin of the colonization event is still a matter of debate, it is certain that Late Glacial and Early Holocene Scotland would have comprised a mosaic of habitats that could have supported a variety of foodways. The wide range of resources exploited by Holocene foragers in Scotland is attested in the faunal assemblages recovered from coastal shell midden sites. Diversity is most apparent in aquatic resources; foods include fish, shellfish, sea mammals, echinoderms, brachyurans and algae. However, a full appreciation of the foods consumed by Mesolithic foragers and their relative importance can only be gained from consideration of the evidence provided by faunal remains, and the results of stable isotope analyses of human and animal remains, in combination with evidence provided by ethnographic and ethno-historical records of foraging groups. This paper presents a synthesis of data from across Scotland and seeks to provide new insights into the variability of Mesolithic diets.

The Scottish Mesolithic – Reconstructing Diet

The Scottish Mesolithic has been the focus of enquiry since the mid-nineteenth century (e.g. Dalrymple 1866; Mann 1908); many sites have been identified and excavated (e.g. Mellars 1987; Wickham-Jones 1990). However, it is only at shell midden sites that organic remains have been preserved in abundance (Figs. 8.1, 8.2). For this reason interpretations of the relative importance of different foods in the diet of Scottish Mesolithic populations have been based on analyses of the faunal and floral remains and the limited range of artefacts recovered from a small number of coastal shell midden sites. Initial investigations of these sites were undertaken in the late nineteenth and early twentieth centuries (e.g. Anderson 1895, 1898; Bishop 1914) though by modern standards the documentation of the faunal and floral remains recovered in those excavations was poor. From the limited accounts available it is evident that shellfish, fish and sea mammals were plentiful, whereas the remains of terrestrial mammals were relatively restricted in range and abundance. Excavations on Oronsay in the 1970s enhanced understanding of economic practices in the final stage of the Scottish Mesolithic

Food Diversity in Mesolithic Scotland

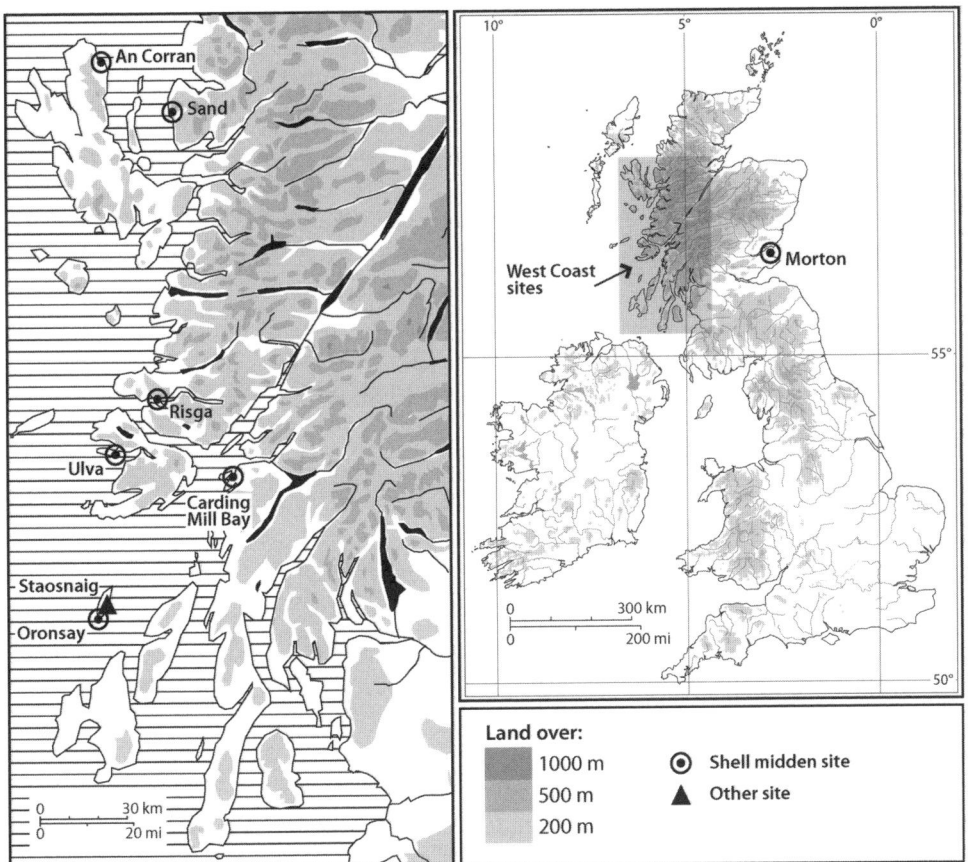

Figure 8.1. Sites mentioned in the text.

(Mellars 1987); however archaeozoological and archaeobotanical remains reflect not just potential foods but also resources harvested for use as raw material and fuel. It is not always possible to distinguish between food and non-food use in archaeological assemblages but the application of stable isotope analysis to the reconstruction of past human diet has, to some extent, addressed this issue.

The Stable Isotope Revolution and the Scottish Mesolithic: Problems and Perspectives

It has become commonplace to examine the bone chemistry of archaeological populations to provide information on 'lifetime' diet (Schwarcz and Schoeninger 1991). Stable isotope analysis has the further advantage of informing on the range of foods that were actually consumed by an individual. Analysis of collagen from human remains in

Figure 8.2. Radiocarbon determinations of sites mentioned in text (from Ashmore 2004).

Site	Lab Ref.	Material	14C age BP*	Calibrated date BC (1σ)
An Corran	OxA-4994	bone, artefact	7590±90	6600-6230
	AA-27746	bone, ruminant	6420±75	5480-5340
	AA-29316	bone, artefact	6215±60	5300-5060
	AA-27746	bone, animal	6420±75	5530-5210
	AA-29316	bone, artefact	6215±60	5310-4990
	AA-29315	bone, artefact	5190±55	4220-3800
Caisteal nan Gillean I (Oronsay)	Q-3008	charcoal	6190±80	5320-4850
	Q-3007	charcoal	6120±80	5290-4800
	Q-3009	charcoal	6035±70	5210-4720
	Q-3010	charcoal	5485±50	4540-4040
	SRR-1458b	marine shells	5485±80	4500-4050
	Q-3011	charcoal	5450±50	4500-3990
	SRR-1458a	charcoal	4750±180	4300-2800
Caisteal nan Gillean II (Oronsay)	Q-1355	charcoal	5460±65	4500-4000
	Birm-347	charcoal	5450±140	4750-3800
	Birm-348	marine shells	5445±435	5400-3100
	Birm-348B	marine shells	5315±200	4550-3650
	Birm-348C	marine shells	5165±200	4450-3500
	Birm-346	charcoal	5150±380	5300-2600
Carding Mill Bay I	OxA-3740	antler, artefact	5190±85	4230-3790
	GU-2796	charcoal	5060±50	3970-3710
	GU-2899	marine shell	5035±65	3970-3660
	GU-2898	marine shell	5005±70	3960-3660
	GU-2797	charcoal	4980±50	3940-3650
	OxA-7664	bone, human	4830±45	3710-3520
	OxA-7663	bone, human	4800±50	3700-3380
	OxA-3739	bone, artefact	4765±65	3660-3370
	OxA-7665	bone, human	4690±40	3630-3360

* The dates on marine shells have been corrected for the marine reservoir effect.

Figure 8.2. Radiocarbon determinations of sites mentioned in text (from Ashmore 2004).

Site	Lab Ref.	Material	14C age BP*	Calibrated date BC (1σ)
Cnoc Coig (Oronsay)	Birm-326X	marine shell	7205±215	6500-5650
	Q-3006	charcoal	5675±60	4690-4360
	Q-3005	charcoal	5650±60	4670-4350
	Q-1353	charcoal	5645±80	4800-4250
	Q-1354	charcoal	5535±140	4800-3950
	Q-1351	charcoal	5495±75	4550-4000
	Q-1352	charcoal	5430±130	4700-3800
Cnoc Sligeach (Oronsay)	Birm-463I	marine shells	7815±240	7500-6200
	Birm-463m	marine shells	6805±185	6100-5350
	Birm-464I	marine shells	6505±230	5850-4850
	Birm-464m	marine shells	6435±270	5900-4700
	Birm-462m	marine shells	5985±230	5500-4300
	GX-1904	bones, animal	5755±180	5300-4000
	Birm-465I	marine shell	5605±215	4950-3950
	Birm-465m	marine shell	5495±215	4800-3800
	Birm-462I	marine shells	5445±140	4800-3800
	BM-670	charcoal	5426±159	4700-3900
Morton B	Q-981	charcoal	6382±120	5650-4850
	Q-988	charcoal	6147±90	5400-4700
	Q-928	charcoal	6115±110	5500-4600
	OxA-4612	bone, artefact	5790±80	4830-4450
	OxA-4611	bone, artefact	5475±60	4460-4140
	OxA-4610	bone, artefact	5180±70	4230-3790
Priory Midden (Oronsay)	Q-3001	charcoal	5870±50	5000-4450
	Q-3000	charcoal	5825±50	4950-4400
	Q-3002	charcoal	5717±50	4800-4340
	Q-3003	charcoal	5510±50	4600-4000
	Q-3004	charcoal	5470±70	4550-4000

* The dates on marine shells have been corrected for the marine reservoir effect.

Figure 8.2. Radiocarbon determinations of sites mentioned in text (from Ashmore 2004).

Site	Lab code	Material	Date BP	Cal BC
Risga	OxA-2023	bone, artefact	6000±90	5250-4600
	OxA-3737	bone, artefact	5875±65	4910-4550
Sand	OxA-10152	bone, artefact	8470±90	7750-7200
	OxA-10384	bone, artefact	7855±60	7050-6500
	OxA-10175	bone, artefact	7825±55	7050-6450
	OxA-9343	charcoal	7765±50	6680-6460
	OxA-9281	bone, artefact	7715±55	6650-6440
	OxA-9282	bone, artefact	7545±50	6470-6240
	OxA-9280	antler	7520±50	6460-6240
	OxA-10176	bone, artefact	6605±50	5630-5470
	OxA-10177	bone, artefact	6485±55	5540-5320
Staosnaig	AA-21627	charred hazelnut shells	8110±60	7330-6830
	AA-21624	charred hazelnut shells	7935±55	7050-6650
	AA-21621	charred hazelnut shell	7780±55	6750-6460
	AA-21625	charred hazelnut shell	7780±55	6750-6460
	AA-21619	charred hazelnut shell	7760±55	6690-6460
	Q-3278	charred hazelnut shells	7720±110	7050-6250
	AA-21623	charred hazelnut shell	7665±55	6640-6420
	AA-21622	charred hazelnut shell	7660±55	6640-6410
	AA-26227	charred hazelnut shell	7420±65	6420-6090
	AA-21620	charred hazelnut shell	7040±55	6020-5780
	AA-21629	charred hazelnut shell	5415±60	4360-4040
Ulva Cave	GU-2704	soil, humic acid	7800±160	7150-6550
	GU-2600	limpet shells	7655±80	6660-6260
	GU-2601	limpet shells	7615±80	6640-6250
	OxA-3738	antler, artefact	5750±70	4780-4450
	GU-2602	limpet shells	5685±80	4710-4350
	GU-2603	limpet shells	5930±70	4550-4160
	GU-2707	charcoal	4990±60	3950-3650

* The dates on marine shells have been corrected for the marine reservoir effect.

the midden at Cnoc Coig on Oronsay confirmed the importance of marine resources for at least some of the Mesolithic population of Scotland (Richards and Mellars 1998). Analysis of a single bone from the roughly contemporaneous site of Caisteal nan Gillean II, also on Oronsay, produced a slightly different result (Fig. 8.3), which was interpreted as representing a diet based on a mix of terrestrial and marine resources. It was suggested that the individual was an incomer to the island, possibly reflecting extra-local marriage practices (Richards and Mellars 1998, 183).

Although stable isotope analysis has undeniably revolutionized dietary reconstruction, the technique has significant limitations that, when combined with the shortcomings of the archaeological record, restrict the validity of palaeodietary reconstructions for the Scottish Mesolithic. For instance, it is well known that the nitrogen and carbon incorporated into bone collagen are derived from dietary protein (Vogel and van der Merwe 1977). It follows that the lipid and carbohydrate components of diets are effectively 'invisible' in individuals with a moderate to high protein intake (Ambrose and Norr 1993) – i.e. most European Mesolithic populations. Palaeodietary reconstructions based on stable isotope analyses of human bone collagen may not, therefore, reflect the full extent of dietary diversity. Furthermore, the interpretation of stable isotope results in the absence of a comparative database of contemporaneous foodstuffs is problematic because of the observed spatial and temporal variation in the stable isotope signals of potential foods (e.g. Ambrose 1991; Heaton 1999). Finally, there is a lack of suitable human remains for analysis: no formal burials of Mesolithic date have been discovered in Scotland. The bones analyzed by Richards and Mellars (1998) represent a very small sample of the Mesolithic population (possibly as few as three individuals), from sites that are both geographically and temporally restricted. Given the myriad problems associated with the reconstruction of Mesolithic foodways in Scotland a full appreciation of the diversity of foods exploited is unlikely to be realized in the near future. However, a preliminary picture of dietary diversity may be derived from a consideration of faunal and floral remains in archaeological sites, supplemented by ethnographic evidence.

Site	Sample	$\delta^{13}C$	$\delta^{15}N$
Casteal nan Gillean II	metatarsal	-15.8	14.6
Cnoc Coig	adult female? right clavicle	-13.2	14.5
Cnoc Coig	adult male left clavicle	-12.3	16.0
Cnoc Coig	adult metacarpal	-12.0	15.7
Cnoc Coig	adult metacarpal	-12.0	17.0
Cnoc Coig	adult frontal	-13.6	15.2

Figure 8.3. Oronsay human bone collagen stable isotope values (from Richards and Mellars 1998, table 1).

Food Diversity in the Scottish Mesolithic

Direct comparison of the diversity of resources exploited at each of the midden sites is hampered by a number of factors, including variability in the size, duration and preservation of the middens; excavation and sampling strategies; processing techniques and also non-publication of specialist reports. Generally, however, the faunal and floral remains recovered from Mesolithic shell middens on both the east and west coasts of Scotland suggest significant dietary diversity which must, in part, reflect the resources available in distinctive micro-environments as well as individual or group preferences in resource selection.

Aquatic Resources

At each of the sites considered in this paper aquatic food remains formed a significant proportion of the midden deposits. The range of species represented is variable. For example, at Ulva Cave 36 distinct taxa of shellfish have been identified (Pickard and Bonsall in press); at Morton the shellfish assemblage was similarly diverse with 37 taxa recorded (Coles 1971). By contrast at An Corran, Skye, 14 genera were recovered from Early to Middle Holocene deposits (Pickard and Bonsall in press) and at Sand, Applecross, only eight taxa were recorded (Milner 2009).

Fish are reported to be abundant at all sites but, unfortunately, detailed reports of the fish bone assemblages are scarce. With the exception of Sand (Parks and Barrett 2009), species diversity is generally limited, but this may reflect publication standards rather than procurement specialization. Species from the cod family (Gadidae) are recorded at all sites for which accounts are available, and saithe (*Pollachius virens*) dominates the ichthyofauna recovered at the Oronsay sites (Anderson 1895, 1898; Connock et al. 1993; Mellars and Payne 1971; Mellars and Wilkinson 1980).

Sea mammals were recovered at the Oronsay sites, Risga in Loch Sunart, and Sand (Anderson 1898; Grigson and Mellars 1987; Lacaille 1954; Parks and Barrett 2009). Finds include the very large rorqual (*Balaenoptera* spp.), and several smaller species – seals (Phocidae) and dolphin or porpoise (*Delphinus delphis/Phocaena phocaena*).

Brachyurans, or true crabs, are present in most of the middens. Generally, where data are available, the presence of edible, swimming and green shore crab is reported (e.g. Anderson 1898; Coles 1971; Lacaille 1954). At Ulva Cave at least six species of crab were identified (Pickard and Bonsall 2009). Lobster (*Homarus gammarus*) was recorded at the Oronsay sites (Mellars and Payne 1971). Fine sieving of midden samples from Ulva Cave also recovered fragments of tests belonging to sea urchins or Echinoidea (Pickard and Bonsall 2009).

Other resources foraged on the shore include aquatic algae, inferred from the presence of small shellfish that live on seaweed but would have little food or decorative value. The seaweeds may have been harvested as food, fuel, or for medicinal properties (e.g. Banga 2002; Turner and Clifton 2006). Such shellfish species were particularly abundant at Ulva Cave (Pickard and Bonsall in press). This may indicate a particular emphasis on seaweed collection at this site, but more likely reflects the sampling strategy adopted (Pickard and Bonsall in press).

Terrestrial Resources

Although remains of terrestrial mammals can be common in shell midden sites, they are generally characterized by low species diversity – 15 species/genera have been identified in Mesolithic deposits. Red deer (*Cervus elaphus*) and wild boar (*Sus scrofa*) are the most commonly recorded large mammals (Kitchener et al. 2004). Otter (*Lutra lutra*) was identified at Risga and at all five Oronsay shell midden sites excavated by Mellars (Lacaille 1954; Mellars 1987). Other 'fur' species identified in the Scottish shell middens include badger (*Meles meles*), fox (*Vulpes vulpes*), marten (*Martes* spp.), and Felidae (Anderson 1895, 1898; Lacaille 1954; Parks and Barrett 2009). Several species of small mammals such as vole (*Microtus agrestis*), common shrew (*Sorex araneus*) and bat (Chiroptera) may have been gathered as food, commensal with human activity, or were simply later intrusions into Mesolithic contexts.

A wide range of bird species were identified at Morton with seabirds such as razorbill (*Alca torda*), and cormorant (*Phalacrocorax carbo*), comprising a significant proportion of the assemblage; however the relative abundance of the remains was not quantified (Coles 1971). Similar diversity of bird species is recorded at Risga although a distinct range of seabirds, including the now extinct great auk (*Pinguinus impennis*), were documented (Lacaille 1954). The majority of the species are seabirds that nest on cliffs or inhabit inshore waters.

The remains of terrestrial food plants from Scottish shell middens are not widely reported. Although carbonized hazelnut (*Corylus avellana*) shells are documented from most of the middens, few other food plants have been identified. Corn spurry (*Spergula arvensis*), stitchwort (*Stellaria* spp.), chickweed (*Stellaria media*), fat hen (*Chenopodium album*) and knotgrass (*Polygonum aviculare*), consistent features of the stomach contents of Iron Age bog bodies (e.g. Harild et al. 2007), were identified at Morton and/or Carding Mill Bay I (Coles 1971; Connock et al. 1993), although it is not clear if the sequence at Carding Mill Bay I extends back into the Mesolithic (Bonsall and Smith 1992; Bartosiewicz et al. 2010). Intensive use of plants is implied by the evidence from Staosnaig on the island of Colonsay, adjacent to Oronsay. Here the remains of an estimated 120–330,000 'roasted' hazelnuts were recovered from pit features, and lesser celandine (*Ranunculus ficaria*) also appears to have been collected as food, but no shell middens were recorded (Mithen et al. 2001).

Discussion

Consideration of the behavioural ecology of the shellfish and crustacean species identified may indicate harvesting strategies. Two genera, limpet (*Patella* spp.) and periwinkle (*Littorina* spp.), dominate the west-coast midden assemblages. The relative abundance of the major species identified at each of the sites generally reflects that of modern shore populations in the region (Little and Kitching 1996). However, the virtual absence of dogwhelk (*Nucella lapillus*), one of the most common carnivorous gastropods on modern shores, at An Corran may reflect shore ecology or cultural practices (Pickard and Bonsall in press). Overall, the evidence points to the adoption of least-effort harvesting strategies at most sites (Connock et al. 1993; Pickard and Bonsall in press). The majority of the species identified are epifaunal littoral species, i.e. species that live on the substrate surface and occupy tidal regions of the shore. They are most readily collected at low tide with little or no equipment.

Infaunal and sublittoral shellfish and crustacean species that live below low water and/or buried in the substrate are rare at midden sites on the west coast of Scotland, although a recent marine survey attests to their abundance in coastal waters (McKay 1992). Some species such as the king scallop (*Pecten maximus*) were collected not as food but as empty shells for use as raw material (Russell et al. 1995).

Infaunal bivalves are more characteristic of Mesolithic shell middens on the east coast of Scotland, where soft shorelines are prevalent. In traditional and commercial shellfisheries bivalves are the most highly valued shellfish in terms of palatability and quantity of flesh (e.g. Gosling 2003). In the Late Mesolithic midden at Morton in Fife one of the most abundant shellfish was Baltic tellin (*Macoma balthica*). Its presence implies foraging in low salinity coastal environments (Coles 1971) consistent with the evidence of extensive estuarine areas near the site around the time of midden accumulation (Chisholm 1971).

'Least effort' or 'little equipment' strategies appear to extend to fishing activities at several of the middens. Specialized fishing equipment is rare in Scottish Mesolithic contexts. However, fishing strategies may be inferred from the species recovered and their size distribution. Gadids (Gadidae), wrasse (Labridae) and flatfish (Pleuronectidae) are most vulnerable to line fishing (Pickard 2002). One of the few finds of fishing gear attributed to the Scottish Mesolithic is a possible bone fishhook from Risga (Morrison 1980: plate XIV). The simplest forms of line fishing do not require hooks. Successful fishing with baited lines, colloquially known as 'bobbing', for small near-shore fish is widely practised (e.g. Kroeber and Barrett 1962). Migratory species are frequently the focus of specialized large-scale traditional fisheries where they are taken with stationary fishing equipment (e.g. Watanabe 1973). For instance European eel (*Anguilla anguilla*) was recovered at Carding Mill Bay I, Oban (Connock et al. 1993) and at Sand (Parks and Barrett 2009). Bones of salmonid (*Salmo* sp.) and the Atlantic sturgeon (*Acipenser sturio*) were found in the shell midden at Morton (Coles 1971). However the evidence from Scotland is insufficient to demonstrate scheduled exploitation with mass-capture fishing gear since migratory species are also susceptible to capture with simple hook and line.

The remains of large terrestrial animals are suggestive of transport to midden sites for use as raw material rather than food residue. Anderson (1895, 1898) proposed that the splinters of large terrestrial mammal bones recovered from the Obanian middens

Food Diversity in Mesolithic Scotland

indicated use primarily for the manufacture of artefacts such as pins, barbed bone points and bevel-ended tools. Grigson and Mellars (1987) noted that the most abundant elements in the red deer assemblage from Cnoc Coig were fragments of antler attesting to industrial use, while the main meat-bearing bones of wild boar were absent from the assemblage. There was no unequivocal evidence for the consumption of either species at the site (Grigson and Mellars 1987). It has been suggested that terrestrial mammals were economically important as a source of raw material to many recent and prehistoric coastal foragers, but did not necessarily comprise a significant component of the diet (Hodgetts and Rahemtullah 2001).

Sea mammals may have been a more important source of food than terrestrial mammals at certain sites. For example, seals dominate the mammalian assemblage at Cnoc Coig, although their remains were not numerous (Grigson and Mellars 1987). Both harbour seal (*Phoca vitulina*) and grey seal (*Halichoerus grypus*), which are commonly found in near-shore waters, could have been sought on haul-outs and skerries (Grigson and Mellars 1987). By contrast rorqual (*Balaenoptera* spp.), which was recorded at Risga (Lacaille 1954), is generally an open-sea species. Fin whale (*Balaenoptera physalus*), which was tentatively identified at Caisteal nan Gillean I and Priory Midden (Grigson and Mellars 1987), is seldom encountered in inshore waters. As there is no clear evidence for subsistence fishing in open-sea waters (Pickard and Bonsall 2004) and given the size of the fin whale and other rorquals, it is likely that Mesolithic groups exploited occasional stranded animals on the shore – a practice widely documented historically (e.g. Olsen 1999).

Smaller terrestrial mammals and seabirds prized for their furs and skins in historically documented forager societies (e.g. Oakes 1991) are relatively common in the middens. While these species may have been taken primarily for their furs or skins, the meat may have been consumed. Similarly, although likely used for food (e.g. Grigson and Mellars 1987), seals and other sea mammals could also have been exploited for fur, skin and intestines, which have traditionally been used in the manufacture of waterproof clothing and vessels (e.g. Lantis 1938). This is supported by Grigson and Mellars' (1987) observation that skin and blubber were extracted from very young seals at Cnoc Coig, whereupon the carcasses were discarded.

Conclusion

This review of the evidence from coastal shell middens in Scotland allows us to draw a number of general conclusions about the food acquisition strategies of Mesolithic people. It is now clear that a wide diversity of food resources were exploited by Mesolithic maritime hunter-gatherers: although the shell middens tend to be dominated by the remains of marine molluscs and fish, there is often also evidence for the exploitation of crabs, echinoderms, marine mammals and seaweed, as well as terrestrial animals and plants. Marine mammal remains occur in some middens but the frequency and pattern of their occurrence is indicative of opportunistic exploitation. The role of terrestrial resources is equivocal. Remains of edible plants are not widely reported, but they were only systematically recovered at a few sites. Terrestrial mammals appear to have been extensively exploited as a source of raw material, but there is no conclusive evidence that they constituted a dietary staple in coastal regions. Notwithstanding the overall diversity of food remains represented in Mesolithic shell middens in Scotland, there is significant variability between sites in terms of the range of species exploited. It is currently difficult to judge to what extent this reflects variations in local ecology, food preferences or sampling strategies and it seems likely that the issue will only be resolved with further detailed analyses.

References

Ambrose, S.H. 1991. 'Effects of diet, climate and physiology on nitrogen isotope abundances in terrestrial foodwebs', *Journal of Archaeological Science* 18, 293–317.

—— and Norr, L. 1993. 'Experimental evidence for the relationship of the carbon isotope ratios of whole diet and dietary protein to those of bone collagen and carbonate', in Lambert, J.B. and Grupe, G. (eds) *Prehistoric Human Bone: Archaeology at the Molecular Level* (Berlin), 1–37.

Anderson, J. 1895. 'Notice of a cave recently discovered at Oban, containing human remains, and a refuse-heap of shells and bones of animals, and stone and bone implements', *Proceedings of the Society of Antiquaries of Scotland* 29, 211–230.

—— 1898. 'Notes on the contents of a small cave or rock-shelter at Druimvargie, Oban; and of three shell-mounds in Oronsay', *Proceedings of the Society of Antiquaries of Scotland* 32, 298-313.

Ashmore, P. 2004. 'A date list for early foragers in Scotland', in Saville, A. (ed.) *Mesolithic Scotland and its Neighbours* (Edinburgh), 95–157.

Banga, B. 2002. 'Seaweed: used for everything from fertilizer to food', *Sea Technology* 43, 15–22.

Bartosiewicz, L., Zapata, L. and Bonsall, C. 2010. 'A tale of two shell middens: the natural *versus* the cultural in "Obanian" deposits at Carding Mill Bay, Oban, western Scotland', in VanDerwarker, A.M. and Peres, T.M. (eds) *Integrating Zooarchaeology and Paleoethnobotany: A Consideration of Issues, Methods, and Cases* (New York), 205–225.

Bishop, A.H. 1914. 'An Oransay shell-mound – a Scottish pre-Neolithic site', *Proceedings of the Society of Antiquaries of Scotland* 48, 52–108.

Bonsall, C. and Smith, C.A. 1992. 'New AMS ^{14}C dates for antler and bone artifacts from Great Britain', *Mesolithic Miscellany* 13(2), 28–34.

Chisholm, J.I. 1971. 'The stratigraphy of the Post-glacial marine transgression in N.E. Fife', *Bulletin of the Geological Survey of Great Britain* 37, 91–107.

Coles, J.M. 1971. 'The early settlement of Scotland: excavations at Morton, Fife', *Proceedings of the Prehistoric Society* 38, 284–366.

Connock, K.D., Finlayson, B. and Mills, C.M. 1993. 'Excavation of a shell midden at Carding Mill Bay, near Oban, Scotland', *Glasgow Archaeological Journal* 17, 25–38.

Dalrymple, C.E. 1866. 'Notes of the excavation of two shell-mounds on the eastern coast of Aberdeenshire', *Proceedings of the Society of Antiquaries of Scotland* 6, 423–426.
Gosling, E. 2003. *Bivalve Molluscs: Biology, Ecology and Culture* (Oxford).
Grigson, C. and Mellars, P. 1987. 'The mammalian remains from the middens', in Mellars, P. (ed.) *Excavations on Oronsay. Prehistoric Human Ecology on a Small Island* (Edinburgh), 243–289.
Harild, J.A., Robinson, D.E. and Hudlebusch, J. 2007. 'New analyses of Grauballe Man's gut contents', in Asingh, P. and Lynnerup, N. (eds) *Grauballe Man. An Iron Age Bog Body Revisited* (Moesgaard), 154–187.
Heaton, T.H.E. 1999. 'Spatial, species and temporal variations in the $^{13}C/^{12}C$ ratios of C_3 plants: implications for palaeodiet', *Journal of Archaeological Science* 26, 637–649.
Hodgetts, L. and Rahemtulla, F. 2001. 'Land and sea: the use of terrestrial mammal bones in coastal hunter-gatherer communities', *Antiquity* 75, 56–62.
Kitchener, A.C., Bonsall, C. and Bartosiewicz, L. 2004. 'Missing mammals from Mesolithic middens: a comparison of the fossil and archaeological records', in Saville, A. (ed.) *Mesolithic Scotland and its Nearest Neighbours: the Early Holocene Prehistory of Scotland its British and Irish Context and some Northern European Perspectives* (Edinburgh), 73–82.
Kroeber, A.L. and Barrett, S.A. 1962. *Fishing Among the Indians of Northwestern California*, (Berkley).
Lacaille, A.D. 1954. *The Stone Age in Scotland* (London).
Lantis, M. 1938. 'The mythology of Kodiak Island, Alaska', *The Journal of American Folklore* 51, 123–172.
Little, C. and Kitching, J. A. 1996. *The Biology of Rocky Shores* (Oxford).
Mann, L.M. 1908. 'Notices (1) of a pottery churn from the Island of Coll, with Remarks on Hebridean pottery; and (2) of a workshop for flint implements in Wigtownshire', *Proceedings of the Society of Antiquaries of Scotland* 42, 326–329.
McKay, D. W. 1992. *Report on a Survey Around Scotland of Potentially Exploitable Burrowing Bivalve Molluscs* (Aberdeen, Fisheries Research Services Collaborative/Contract Reports 01/92).
Mellars, P. 1987. *Excavations on Oronsay. Prehistoric Human Ecology on a Small Island* (Edinburgh).
—— and Payne, S. 1971. 'Excavation of two Mesolithic shell middens on the Island of Oronsay (Inner Hebrides)', *Nature* 231, 387–398.
—— and Wilkinson, M.R. 1980. 'Fish otoliths as indicators of seasonality in prehistoric shell middens: the evidence from Oronsay (Inner Hebrides)', *Proceedings of the Prehistoric Society* 46, 19–44.
Milner, N. 2009. 'Mesolithic middens and marine molluscs, procurement and consumption of shellfish at the site of Sand', in Hardy, K. and Wickham-Jones, C. (eds) *Mesolithic and Later Sites around the Inner Sound, Scotland: The Work of the Scotland's First Settlers Project 1998–2004.* http://www.sair.org.uk/sair31/
Mithen, S., Finlay, N., Carruthers, W., Carter, S. and Ashmore, P. 2001. 'Plant use in the Mesolithic: evidence from Staosnaig, Isle of Colonsay, Scotland', *Journal of Archaeological Science* 28, 223–234.
Morrison, A. 1980. *Early Man in Britain and Ireland* (London).
Oakes, J. 1991. 'Environmental factors influencing bird-skin clothing production', *Arctic and Alpine Research* 23, 71–79.
Olsen, J. 1999. 'Killing methods and equipment in the Faroese Pilot Whale Hunt. Translation of "Om avlivningsmetoder og udstyr for færøsk grindefangst"', (Greenland, Paper presented at the NAMMCO Workshop on Hunting Methods, Nuuk, Greenland, 9–11 February 1999).
Parks, R. and Barrett, J. 2009 'The Zooarchaeology of Sand', in Hardy, K. and Wickham-Jones, C. (eds) *Mesolithic and Later Sites around the Inner Sound, Scotland: The Work of the Scotland's First Settlers Project 1998–2004.* http://www.sair.org.uk/sair31/.
Pickard, C. 2002. *Fishing in Mesolithic Europe*, unpublished PhD thesis, University of Edinburgh.
—— and Bonsall, C. 2004. 'Deep sea fishing in the European Mesolithic: fact or fantasy?', *European Journal of Archaeology* 7, 273–290.
—— and Bonsall, C. 2009. 'Some observations on the Mesolithic crustacean assemblage from Ulva Cave, Inner Hebrides, Scotland', in Burdukiewicz, J.M., Cyrek, K., Dyczek, P. and Szymczak, K. (eds) *Understanding the Past. Papers Offered to Stefan K. Kozłowski* (Warsaw), 305–313.
—— and Bonsall, C. in press. 'Mesolithic and Early Neolithic shell middens in western Scotland; a comparative

analysis of shellfish exploitation patterns', in Roksandic, M., Mendonça, S., Eggers, S., Burchell, M. and Klokler, D. (eds) *The Cultural Dynamics of Shell Middens and Shell Mounds: A Worldwide Perspective* (Albuquerque).

Richards, M.P. and Mellars, P. 1998. 'Stable isotopes and the seasonality of the Oronsay middens', *Antiquity* 72, 178–184.

Ritchie, G. and Ritchie, A. 1991. *Scotland: Archaeology and Early History* (Edinburgh).

Russell, N., Bonsall, C. and Sutherland, D.G. 1995. 'The exploitation of marine molluscs in the Mesolithic of western Scotland: evidence from Ulva Cave, Inner Hebrides', in Fischer, A. (ed.) *Man and Sea in the Mesolithic* (Oxford), 273–288.

Schwarcz, H. and Schoeninger, M. 1991. 'Stable isotope analyses in human nutritional ecology', *Yearbook of Physical Anthropology* 34, 283–321.

Turner, N.J. and Clifton, H. 2006. 'The forest and the seaweed: gitga'at seaweed, traditional ecological knowledge, and community survival', in Menzies, C.R. (ed.) *Traditional Ecological Knowledge and Natural Resource Management* (Lincoln), 66–86.

Vogel, J.C. and van der Merwe, N.J. 1977. 'Isotopic evidence for early maize cultivation in New York State', *American Antiquity* 42, 238–242.

Watanabe, H. 1973 (rev. ed.). *The Ainu Ecosystem* (Seattle).

Wickham-Jones, C. 1990. *Rhum: Mesolithic and Later Sites at Kinloch* (Edinburgh).

Recognition and Interpretation of a Singular Late Bronze Age Animal Sacrifice Event at Kilise Tepe, Turkey

Peter R. W. Popkin, British Institute at Ankara

Many Hittite texts describing rituals, festivals and feasting events involving animal sacrifice have been recovered and translated, informing researchers about ceremonial and ritual practice in Hittite Anatolia. The interpretation of these texts is often focused on the role of cult and priesthood in society, the nature and timing of particular festivals or the understanding of deities and their relationship with humans (cf. Beckman 1983, 1990; Gurney 1976; Miller 2004; Singer 1983). Recently the role of the animals themselves has become a focus of study (Collins 1990, 2002, 2006a, 2006b). In particular, Mouton (2004, 2005, 2007, 2008, in press) has investigated the treatment of animal carcasses after death and how different body-parts were used as offerings.

Zooarchaeology has the potential to confirm and extend textual interpretations of animal use during Hittite rituals, festivals and feasting events through an analysis of skeletal remains and their depositional context. To date, few zooarchaeological reports have been published from Anatolian sites dating to the Late Bronze Age–Early Iron Age (hereafter LBA and EIA) and none of them discusses individual contexts or sacrifice and feasting events (Deniz et al. 1964; von den Driesch and Pöllath 2003; Hongo 1997; 2003, 2004; Howell-Meurs 2001; Ikram 2003; Patterson 1937; Zeder and Arter 1994) with the exception of a reported piglet burial from Yazılıkaya (Hauptmann 1975, 65). Virtually no zooarchaeological evidence exists to confirm or refute textual descriptions of Hittite animal sacrifice and feasting events. This paper aims to redress the imbalance somewhat by providing an analysis of a unique discovery of a disarticulated but almost complete sheep skeleton deposited within a small LBA pit inside a building with ritual associations at Kilise Tepe, Turkey. It is argued that the skeletal remains derive from a sheep sacrificed for a ritual/ceremonial event that was followed by a feasting event. No other evidence for feasting exists at Kilise Tepe, making this deposit particularly important for our understanding of behaviour at the site. The skeletal remains and their depositional context are interpreted via Hittite texts describing rituals involving the sacrifice, consumption and burial of sheep remains in order to reconstruct events surrounding the creation of the deposit. By consistently analysing and publishing small, individual deposits zooarchaeologists can contribute significantly to the study of ritual and feasting.

Kilise Tepe

Kilise Tepe is located in south-central Turkey approximately 40 km inland of the Mediterranean coast in western Cilicia. The site dominates the south-eastern exit from the Mut basin and it controls the local ford of the Göksu river (Postgate 1998, 128). Kilise Tepe is a relatively small mound site measuring approximately 100 x 110m at its summit. Occupation of the site dates from the Early Bronze Age (EBII: 2700–2400 BC) through to the Byzantine period (up to AD 1200), though occupation was not continuous. The sheep burial is associated with Phase IIa/b dating towards the end of the LBA (approximately 1275 BC).

Stele Building

In the north-west sector of the site stands a large (18 x 14m) building, dubbed the stele building after a painted sandstone stele recovered from its central room that has been ascribed ceremonial or ritual (or at the very least, public) function (Postgate and Thomas 2007, 137). The building is not a temple, as such, and many of its rooms served a utilitarian function such as storage of foodstuffs. The large central room (room 3) of the stele building contained a central hearth measuring 80cm in diameter and a diagonally placed table or altar, both of which originally date to phase IIa/b and remained in use through several phases (Postgate and Thomas 2007, 125). Recovered from the triangular area behind the altar were several shells, clay and stone beads and numerous astragali (Postgate and Thomas 2007, 125). A second cache of 99 astragali was recovered, buried beneath the floor of room 7. The painted sandstone stele was recovered from the south-east section of room 3. Ceremonial events taking place in the building would have occurred in this room. The pit (P08/23) containing the sheep deposition (Fig. 9.1) was located in room 2, immediately north of room 3. The pit was contemporary with the initial construction of the building in Phase IIa/b. It was sub-triangular with maximum lengths of approximately 60cm and a maximum depth of approximately 20cm.

Zooarchaeological Evidence

A total of 53 elements were recovered from pit P08/23 belonging to a single animal that was identified as a sheep based on morphological criteria following Boessneck (1969). Morphology of the pelvis (Boessneck 1969) indicated the animal to be male, with ageing data – epiphyseal fusion based on Silver (1969) and dental eruption/wear interpreted according to Payne (1973) and Silver (1969) – suggesting that the individual died at approximately 20–24 months of age. Given that some of the long bones were unfused, the animal may not have reached its full adult size; however, wither height calculations (based on the greatest lengths of the radius, metapodials and calcaneum) estimate a shoulder height of 62–64cm at the time of death (Teichert 1975).

The limited fragmentation and the good preservation of the bones indicate that they were not disturbed or affected by destructive taphonomic processes subsequent

Interpretation of a Singular Late Bronze Age Animal Sacrifice

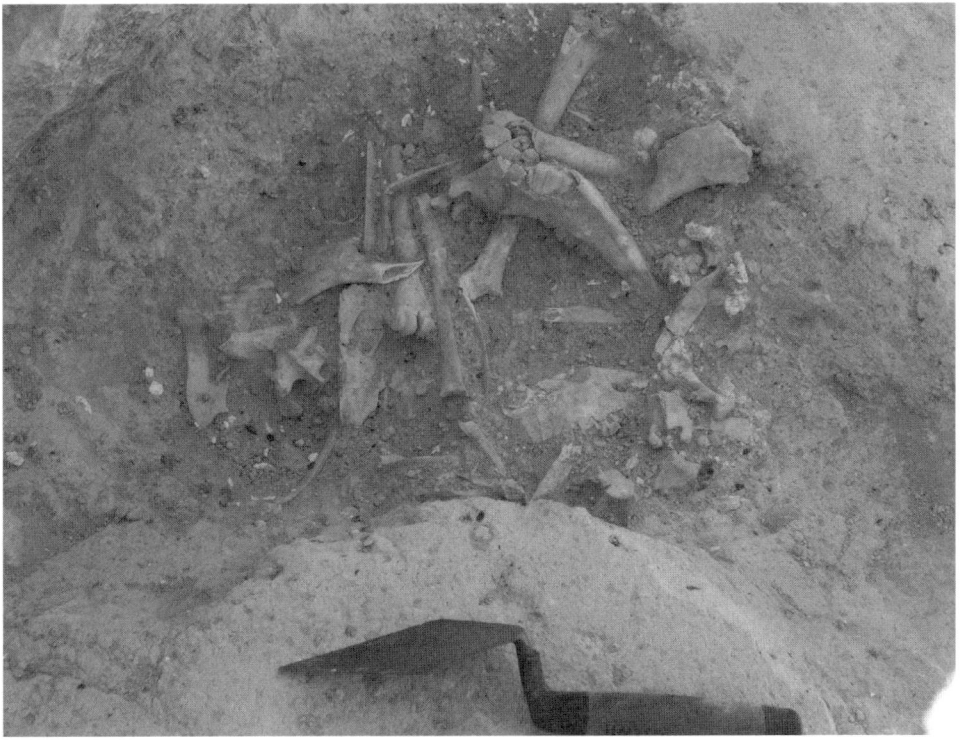

Figure 9.1. Sheep skeleton deposited in pit P08/23 (photograph by the author).

to burial. It is probable that elements not recovered from the pit were not deposited within the pit in the first place. None of the bones shows signs of burning or evidence of gnawing by carnivores.

Elements Recovered

All of the major long bones were recovered (except for the left scapula and right humerus) and most were recovered complete, indicating that the bones were not intentionally broken during the butchery process or subsequently for marrow removal. Most of the left ribs were missing. The bones were deposited in a disarticulated state but local articulations between individual vertebrae and carpals were intact, suggesting that some connective tissue remained. The bones, and possibly other waste from the carcass, were deposited shortly after the animal had been killed. The missing shoulder joints (right humerus, left scapula and most of the left humerus) may have been treated differently from the remainder of the carcass and removed in their entirety prior to filleting. Both astragali were missing and considering the astragali caches recovered at the site it is likely the astragali were intentionally collected from the animal prior to deposition.

Butchery

Disarticulation cut marks, filleting cut marks and heavy chop marks provide evidence for butchering. The chop marks are limited to the axial skeleton and result from a rough sectioning of the spine and pelvis into smaller parcels. Very heavy cut or chop marks are also found on the axis vertebra which result either from enthusiastic slaughtering of the animal by cutting its throat or possibly relate to the decapitation of the animal (Fig. 9.2). Textual evidence indicates it was common Hittite practice to slaughter an animal by cutting its throat in order to bleed the animal (Mouton, in press). Disarticulation cut marks on the limb bones indicate that the carcass was segmented into individual elements in a precise fashion following natural skeletal divisions. Filleting marks indicate that meat was stripped from the skeleton. A series of eleven cut marks on the spine of the right scapula were made during the removal of the origin of the deltoid muscle and filleting marks on the anterio-lateral face of the proximal right femur were made during the removal of the origin of the vastus intermedius muscle.

Deposition

Judging from the lack of archaeological examples, the careful deposition of a sheep carcass in a small pit subsequent to meat removal was an unusual practice in LBA Anatolia. The textual record, on the other hand, indicates that this practice was more common than the archaeology suggests. Reasons for this might include: 1) the practice was occurring off-site, on river-banks for example (see in particular KUB 7.41, below); 2) the pits only occurred in particular buildings (that have yet to be excavated); 3) the

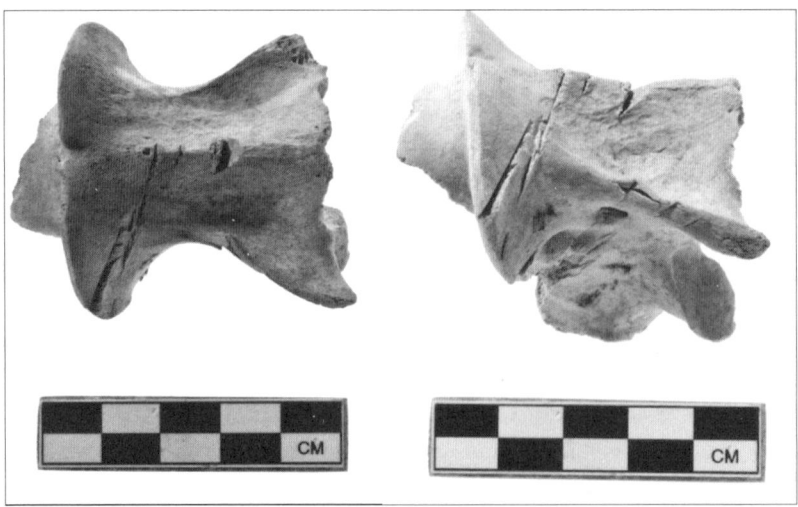

Figure 9.2. Heavily butchered axis vertebrae dorsal (left) and right side (right) views (photographs courtesy Bob Miller).

Interpretation of a Singular Late Bronze Age Animal Sacrifice

pits have been overlooked in past excavations because of their small size and the general lack of interest in zooarchaeological remains; or finally 4) the pits have been excavated but have not been published. To understand more about the use of pits in Hittite ritual and feasting practice we turn now to the textual evidence.

Textual Evidence

Hittites used pits in ritual practice in a variety of ways, including as a channel for communication with chthonic deities; as a means of disposing of impurities by consigning them to the earth as an offering; and as a means of securing the future strength and favour of a structure in the form of a foundation ritual. There is not space here to present all the relevant texts but the selection below illustrates various ritual practices involving both sheep and pits.

Examples of Relevant Texts

1) *Ritual for Drawing of Paths: KUB 15.31* (translation from Collins 2002, 227).

> Promptly he takes a hoe and digs [with it]. Then he takes a pectoral ornament and digs with it. Then he takes a *šatta-*, a spade, and a *huppara-* container, and he clears out [the pit with them]...
>
> He smears the nine pits with blood. Then for the nine pits [there are] nine birds and one lamb. For *ambašši* and *keldi* he offers nine birds and one lamb. He puts one bird in each pit, but the lamb they cut up and put in the first pit.

2) *Ritual to the Underworld Deities for Purifying a House: KUB 7.41* (translation from Collins 2002, 227).

> He goes to the river bank and takes oil, beer, wine, *walhi-*drink, *marnuan-*drink, a cupful [of] each in turn, sweet oil cake, meal, [and] porridge. He holds a lamb and he slaughters it down into a pit (*patteššar*).

3) *Foundation Ritual (For a Temple of the Goddess of the Night): KUB 29.4 and duplicate KBo 8.90* (translation from Mouton 2008, 7; see also Collins 2002, 228).

> When, during the second day, at nightfall, a star twinkles, the ritual patron goes to the temple. He bows down before the deity. The two knives which have been made for the new deity, one takes them. One digs an *āpi-*pit before the table of the deity. One sacrifices a sheep to the deity as *enumašši-*. One slaughters [it] down into the pit.

4) *Foundation Ritual (from the 13th century BCE): KUB 55.26 and Bo 7740* (translation from Ünal 1988, 101).

> Bu[t] to the pillars (sg.) which are on the right and left [side of the owner of the house], to those they sacrifice [sheep] in three different places. Each time, however, they s[ac]rifice one sheep.

In front of the altar, he [the owner of the house] pours beer [and] wine after the blood [offering]. In front of each of the two pillars they libate three times. They place the raw meat [of the sacrificed sheep], the breasts, shoulders, heads, and feet, in front of the altar. The breast, shoulders, heads, [and] feet they place in front of those t[wo] pillars, to [or for] which [animals] have been slaughtered.

5) *Tunnawiya of Hattuša's Ritual of 'Taking off the Earth'*: KUB 55.45 + Bo 69/142ii (translation in Collins 2002, 229).

While they begin digging out the storage pits they drive up a sheep. The old woman consecrates it to the Sun Goddess of the Earth. They slit its throat downward into the storage pit and let its blood flow downward... Then they butcher [the animals] with respect to the heads and feet. While the fat cooks, soldiers dig out a storage pit. When they finish digging it, then they [di]g close by another storage pit. It happens that they join it to the [first] pit. The fat cooks and the entire assembly eats it.

6) *(Winter) Festival for Ishtar of Nineveh*: KUB 10.63 (translation from Collins 2002, 231).

The queen comes forth, and the diviner opens up a pit (*āpi*) before the Storm God *marapši*. The diviner offers one sheep to the Storm God *marapši*, and the diviner cuts its throat downward for the pit. He releases the blood into a cup, which he places on the ground before the Storm God *marapši*. Next the diviner [proceeds] to the raw intestines and heart [of the sacrifice] and cuts off a little. He takes a little blood as well and sets it down into the pit. Then at the top he stops up the pit with thick bread. They carry the sheep forth, and the temple servants cut it up.

Discussion of Texts

None of the available texts specify what becomes of the sheep carcass after it is sacrificed and butchered. Ritual 2 is designed for the purification of a house, or temple, however it takes place next to a river bank and zooarchaeological examples of this ritual will be difficult to find. The description of slaughtering a lamb down into the pit may be referring to letting its blood flow from its neck into the pit at slaughter and not the placement of the carcass in the pit. The house described in ritual 4 can indicate a temple or ceremonial location (Ünal 1988, 102). Architectural elements other than pillars can also receive sacrifices, including walls, hearths, windows, doors, door bolts, columns and altars (Ünal 1988, 103). The pit described in ritual 1 is dug with a hoe and a 'pectoral ornament' and the pits described in rituals 2 and 3 are dug with daggers, suggesting that they are all small, unlined, single-use affairs similar to pit P08/23. The purpose of ritual 5 is to release a suppliant by means of substitution from the influence of the chthonic

Interpretation of a Singular Late Bronze Age Animal Sacrifice

powers and thus to absolve him from his sin and heal him. The ritual describes humans feasting on the sheep that has been consecrated to the Sun Goddess of the Earth. In ritual 6 portions of the intestines, heart and some blood of the sacrificed sheep are placed in the pit. The remainder of the sheep is butchered for human consumption (Collins 2002, 230). The fate of the carcass post-butchery is not stated but it is conceivable it was brought back to the pit, which was only covered by bread, and deposited.

There is no exact parallel between the rituals described in the available texts and the deposit recovered at Kilise Tepe. It is possible, though by no means certain, that the deposit represents the remains of a foundation ritual because the pit dates to the period of the initial construction of the building. It is clear that the meat, and probably the fat and offal, of the sheep have been removed in preparation for a feasting event following the ritual.

Reconstructing the Process of Animal Sacrifice and Consumption

Combining the zooarchaeological and textual evidence allows a tentative reconstruction of the process surrounding the deposition of the sheep bones within the pit in the stele building. Aspects of this reconstruction inevitably rely on extrapolation from known ritual practice and are a matter of conjecture in many instances. The available evidence does not inform us about the feast that occurred subsequent to the slaughter of the animal but it does help us understand the process leading up to the feast and is an example of how zooarchaeological evidence can indirectly indicate feasting events in LBA Anatolia.

1) *Selection*. The animal was selected with a particular ritual/event in mind; species, age, sex and colour may all have been a factor in its selection. Sheep were the animal most frequently offered as sacrifices (Mouton, in press), meaning they were also the animal most frequently eaten during feasts. The age of the animal sacrificed is specified in substitution rituals, where the animal is typically juvenile, but is seldom mentioned in other texts. Sex is not specified for most rituals and may not have been important in this instance but it is taken into consideration during substitution rituals where the sex of the animal usually matches the sex of the devotee (Mouton, in press).
2) *Sanctification*. The animal was brought to the stele building and sanctified through prayer and possibly the ritual burning of incense and/or scented wood. This act bestows a condition of being devoted or sacred upon the animal making it suitable as an offering to a deity. The special deposition of the skeletal material, and possibly other soft-tissue waste, indicates that the whole animal became devoted and not just the meat (*šuppa*) that was subsequently placed before the deity. For a discussion about the ritual devotion of an animal see Mouton (2007).
3) *Preparing the pit*. The pit was dug. The pit's small size, single use and lack of any lining suggest it was dug using small tools as in rituals 1, 2 and 3, above.

4) *Sacrifice*. The animal was sacrificed. The verb most commonly used to describe the slaughter of the animal is *hatt(a)-*, translated as 'prick', 'strike', 'cut open' and 'slit the throat' (Mouton 2007). The act of slaughter represents the moment of destruction of the animal; it is irrevocably sacrificed by its owner. It also facilitates the release of the animal's blood, a powerful ingredient in the ritual process. The sheep was bled out by cutting its jugular veins. The heavy cut marks on the axis likely reflect this act. The animal's blood was collected in a vessel or on bread or allowed to flow into the pit.

5) *Disarticulation*. The animal was disarticulated. Two techniques were used in the process: heavy chopping and precise cutting. Long bones were separated from each other by cutting through the joint; whole joints were not preserved, save perhaps a shoulder joint. The axial skeleton was chopped roughly into smaller parcels. At this stage the left shoulder, left ribs, left shin and offal may have been separated from the rest of the skeleton and prepared as offerings, explaining their absence from the pit. The astragali may also have been collected at this stage for use in future rituals.

6) *Filleting*. Meat was stripped from the bones of the sheep. This meat may not have been offered before the deity but was still sanctified and considered as *šuppa*. It would have been consumed along with the offerings at a subsequent feasting event. If cooked, the meat of the animal was probably boiled rather than roasted as textual evidence indicates roasting is typically reserved for the heart and liver (Mouton 2007). There is no evidence of burning on any of the bones. Meat removal likely occurred prior to cooking. If the bones were boiled, there is every possibility the unfused epiphyseal ends would have become disarticulated which did not occur.

7) *Deposition*. Bones and other waste material were carefully deposited into the pit, reflecting the sanctified nature of the entire animal. It is important to remember the pit was within the stele building and the interment of the sheep in this location carries significance because it differentiates the deposit from common food refuse. The pit was covered.

8) *Offering*. The *šuppa*, made up of meat, offal and possibly fat, were taken into room 3 and placed before the deity, perhaps represented by the stele if it is considered to be a *huwaša* stone. The *šuppa* was left for some period of time before the deity, possibly overnight. There is no zooarchaeological evidence for this action but the ritual associations of the stele building make it possible. On the other hand, if the deposition was the result of a foundation ritual the sheep may not have been offered to a deity at all but rather to an architectural element within the building or to the building itself. It was not necessary to destroy the sacrifice by fire to transmit it to the deity, as was the case in ancient Greece, though complete immolation of sacrifices did occur, particularly in Kizzuwatna rituals (Mouton in press).

9) *Consumption*. The *šuppa* was taken from before the deity and consumed. It was not forbidden for humans to consume *šuppa* after it had been offered to the deity. The *šuppa* that was not offered to the deity would also be consumed at this stage. It is

not clear who would have been able to participate in the feast. Texts describing feasts associated with religious holidays occurring in Hattuša indicate the feasts were restricted to élite members of society including the royal family, palace officials and priests (Mouton in press). Participation at Kilise Tepe, which was a great distance from the Hittite heartland, may have been extended to other social groups.

Conclusions

This paper is an important first step to integrating zooarchaeology with Hittite textual evidence in order to better understand LBA animal sacrifice and feasting events. Engaging in intra-site, deposit-specific zooarchaeological analysis is necessary to corroborate, or perhaps refute, the reality of practices described in texts. This is particularly true at sites, such as Kilise Tepe, located far from the Hittite heartland where most of the texts were recovered. Sites on the edge of empire may have engaged in regional practices not officially recognized or recorded by centrally located scribes. It is also important to record zooarchaeological evidence of ritual behaviour from Anatolian sites so that we may determine regional similarities and differences. This will prove helpful when considering cultural contact across the eastern Mediterranean basin. Finally, the possibility exists that astragali recovered from caches at Kilise Tepe (and possibly elsewhere around the Mediterranean – e.g. Gilmore 1997) were selected from animals that had been sanctified prior to slaughter, enhancing their suitability for use at subsequent ritual events. The same provenance is unlikely to have been required of astragali used in a more profane manner. The analysis performed here demonstrates that zooarchaeology illuminates Anatolian ritual practice and provides evidence of behaviour not preserved in other aspects of the archaeological record.

Acknowledgements
This research was made possible through the support of the British Institute at Ankara and the National Geographic Society.

References
Beckman, G.M. 1983. *Hittite Birth Rituals* (Wiesbaden).
—— 1990. 'The Hittite "Ritual of the Ox" (*CTH* 760.I.2–3)', *Orientalia* 59, 34–55.
Boessneck, J. 1969. 'Osteological differences between sheep (*Ovis aries* Linne) and goat (*Capra hircus* Linne)', in Brothwell, D. and E. Higgs (eds) *Science in Archaeology* (New York), 331–358.
Collins, B.J. 1990. 'The puppy in Hittite ritual', *Journal of Cuneiform Studies* 42, 211–226.
—— 2002. 'Necromancy, fertility and the dark earth: the use of ritual pits in Hittite cult', in Mirecki, P. and M. Meyer (eds) *Magic and Ritual in the Ancient World* (Leiden), 224–241.
—— 2006a. 'A note on some local cults in the time of Tudhaliya IV', in Th.P.J. van den Hout (ed.) *The Life and Times of Hattušili III and Tuthaliya IV* (Leiden), 39–48.
—— 2006b. 'Pigs at the gate: Hittite pig sacrifice in its eastern Mediterranean context', *Journal of Ancient Near Eastern Religions* 6, 155–188.
Deniz, E., Çalışlar, D. and Özgüden, T. 1964. 'Osteological investigations of the animal remains recovered from the excavations of ancient Sardis', *Anatolia* 8, 49–56.

Gilmour, G. 1997. 'The nature and function of astragalus bones from archaeological contexts in the Levant and Eastern Mediterranean', *Oxford Journal of Archaeology* 16, 167–75.

Gurney, O.R. 1976. *Some Aspects of Hittite Religion* (Oxford).

Hauptmann, H. 1975. 'Die architektur: die felsspalte D.', in Bittel, K., Boessneck, J., Damm, B., Güterbock, H.G., Hauptmann, H., Naumann, R. and Schirmer, W. (eds), *Das Hethitishe Felsheiligtum Yazılıkaya* (Berlin), 62–75.

Hongo, H. 1997. *Patterns of Animal Husbandry in Central Anatolia from the 2nd Millennium BC through the Middle Ages: Faunal remains from Kaman-Kalehöyük*. Unpublished PhD Harvard University.

—— 2003. 'Continuity or changes: faunal remains from stratum IId at Kaman-Kalehöyük', in Fischer, B., Genz, H., Jean, É. and Köroğlu, K. (eds) *Identifying Changes: The Transition from Bronze to Iron Ages in Anatolia and its Neighbouring Regions* (Istanbul), 257–270.

—— 2004. 'Transition from the Bronze Age to the Iron Age in Central Anatolia: a view from the faunal remains from Kaman-Kalehöyük', *Anatolian Archaeological Studies* 13, 121–131.

Howell-Meurs, S. 2001. *Early Bronze and Iron Age Animal Exploitation in Northeastern Anatolia: The Faunal Remains from Sos Höyük and Büyüktepe Höyük* (Oxford).

Ikram, S. 2003. 'A Preliminary Study of Zooarchaeological Change between the Bronze and Iron Ages at Kinet Höyük, Hatay', in Fischer, B., Genz, H., Jean, É. and Köroğlu, K. (eds) *Identifying Changes: The Transition from Bronze to Iron Ages in Anatolia and its Neighbouring Regions* (Istanbul), 283–294.

Miller, J.L. 2004. *Studies in the Origins, Development and Interpretation of the Kizzuwatna Rituals* (Wiesbaden).

Mouton, A. 2004. 'Anatomie animale: le festin carné des dieux d'après les textes Hittites I: les membres antérieurs', *Colloquium Anatolicum* 3, 67–92.

—— 2005. 'Anatomie animale: le festin carné des dieux d'après les Textes Hittites II : les membres postérieurs et d'autres parties anatomiques', *Colloquium Anatolicum* 4, 139–154.

—— 2007. 'Anatomie animale: le festin carné des dieux d'après les Textes Hittites III: le traitement des viandes', *Revue Assyriologie et Archéologie Orientale* 101, 81–94.

—— 2008. "Dead of night' in Anatolia: Hittite night rituals', *Religion Compass* 2, 1–17.

—— (in press). 'Le sacrifice animal en Anatolie Hittite', in Rutherford, I. and Hitch, S. (eds), *Violent Commensality: Animal Sacrifice and its Discourses in the Ancient World* (Cambridge).

Patterson, B. 1937. 'Animal remains', in Von Der Osten, H. H. (ed.), *The Alishar Hüyük Seasons of 1930–32 Part III* (Researches in Anatolia IX), 294–309.

Payne, S. 1973. 'Kill-off patterns in sheep and goats: the mandibles from Aşvan Kale', *Anatolian Studies* 23, 281–303.

Postgate, N. 1998. 'Between the plateau and the sea: Kilise Tepe 1994–97', in R. Matthews (ed.) *Ancient Anatolia: Fifty Years Work by the British Institute of Archaeology at Ankara* (Oxford), 127–141.

—— and Thomas, D. 2007. *Excavations at Kilise Tepe 1994–98: From Bronze Age to Byzantine in Western Cilicia*, Volume 1: Text (Cambridge).

Singer, I. 1983. *The Hittite KI.LAM Festival (Part One)* (Wiesbaden).

Silver, I. A. 1969. 'The ageing of the domestic animals', in Brothwell, D. and Higgs, E.S. (eds) *Science in Archaeology* (London), 283–302.

Tiechert, M. 1975. 'Osteometrischeuntersuchungen zur berechnung der widerristhöhe bei schafen', in Clason, A. (ed.) *Archaeological Studies* (Amsterdam), 51–69.

Ünal, A. 1988. '"You should build for eternity" New light on the Hittite architects and their work', *Journal of Cuneiform Studies* 40, 97–106.

von den Driesch, A. and Pöllath, N. 2003. 'Changes from Late Bronze Age to Early Iron Age animal husbandry as reflected in the faunal remains from Büyükkaya/Boğazoköy-Hattuša', in Fischer, B., Genz, H., Jean, É. and Köroğlu, K. (eds) *Identifying Changes: The Transition from Bronze to Iron Ages in Anatolia and its Neighbouring Regions* (Istanbul), 295–300.

Zeder, M.A. and Arter, S.R. 1994. 'Changing patterns of animal utilization at ancient Gordion', *Paléorient* 20, 105–118.

Triple Cups and Bird-Shaped Pottery: Ritualized Feasting-Goods from Norwegian Graves Dating from the First to the Fifth Centuries AD

Christian L. Rødsrud, Museum of Cultural History, University of Oslo

In this article I will focus on two rare groups of pottery from Norwegian graves dating to the first five centuries AD: triple cups and bird-shaped beakers. They are part of an old Scandinavian tradition of drinking rituals with interesting ethnographic parallels connecting them to the feasting practices of sixteenth- and seventeenth-century farming communities. These vessels were not crafted for daily use, but were mostly for drinking on special occasions such as weddings and funerals or for other cultic activities (Gjærder 1975, 181). The vessels point up the life-enhancing qualities of alcohol, brought to humankind by the gods and central to both social and religious life. Both types of objects are loaded with meanings which may be further explored in a wide spectrum of written sources. Linking to recent writings on materiality (Gell 1998; Glørstad and Hedeager 2009; Miller 2005a; Tilley 2006), I will, by the use of analogy, try to show how these artefacts are primary symbols of funerary feasting in early Iron Age society.

Triple Cups

Triple cups consist, as the name implies, of three cups joined together (Fig. 10.1). They are connected internally by small holes at the base, which indicate that the contents of the cups were liquid, flowing from one cup to another. The cups from Hedrum (Fig. 10.1a) and Trålum (Fig. 10.1b) are dated to between the fourth and fifth centuries, while the one from Ula (10.1c) is undated but probably earlier. These finds have close parallels in Norwegian folk woodcarvings of the sixteenth and seventeenth centuries which share exactly the same shape and function as the pottery (Fig. 10.1d–e). Ceremonial use on special occasions like weddings and funerals is documented as their primary function in folk culture up until the nineteenth century, when they were replaced by vessels of other materials which took on new shapes. These vessels were fashioned and embellished with artistic care, while vessels for everyday use have not survived thanks to wear and tear and inferior quality (Christie 1986; Gjærder 1975; Midtun 1921). Worth mentioning as parallels are the 'planetary' pots of Belgic Gaul where triple-faced images appear (Green 1989, 175–176; Lexow 1958, 62).

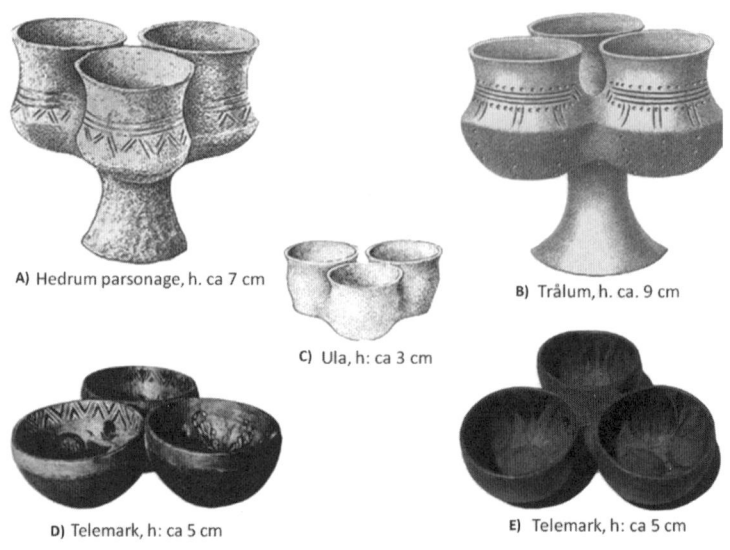

Figure 10.1. Triple cups of pottery (a–c) and wood (d–e), all drawings are out of scale: a) Mus. no. C21408, Hedrum prestegård, Larvik, Vestfold, Norway, AD 350–450 (drawing by Skafft); b) Mus. no. C30491g, Trålum, Fjære, Aust-Agder, Norway, AD 350–450 (drawing by unknown); c) Mus. no. C29860b, Ula, Fredrikstad, Østfold, Norway, probably AD 100–300 (drawing by Tone Strenger); d) Telemark, Norway, eighteenth century (after Gjærder 1975, fig. 242); e) Telemark, Norway, seventeenth/eighteenth century (photograph by the author).

Looking into the literature, it is evident that triple cups were made as early as the late Neolithic and can be found in many cultures until modern times (Gjærder 1975, 122–124, 176–179, 478, 481; Grohne 1932, 32–55; Kaye 1914). Here, I will mainly focus on fully published Norwegian (to some extent other Scandinavian and northern European) examples that can be dated to the first five centuries AD. However, there are many examples known from other parts of Europe, particularly Germany, Britain and Italy (Grohne 1932; Haberey 1953; Kaye 1914; Veeck 1931, 28, Plate C, fig. 25, Plate 17, fig. 12). Interestingly, the southern European finds usually date to the last centuries BC, one or two centuries earlier than those in the north, while most British finds are dated to the Roman period (Bøe 1931,130–131; Fingerlin 1964,32–33; Grohne 1932; Kaye 1914, all with further references). The triple cups are too unusual and complicated to be suitable for ordinary use and bear witness to a highly specialized craft process.

Ritualized Feasting-Goods from Norwegian Graves

The Original Meaning

In Britain triple-cups often go by the name 'fuddling cups', named after a tavern game of the seventeenth century where the drinker was supposed to empty the cup without spilling the contents (Monson-Fitzjohn 1927). This drinking game offers a humorous explanation of the function of the cup, but many such customs can trace their origins to cultic or magical beliefs. The example shows that customs may be context-specific, but I will here try to find clues to the original meaning behind these drinking-vessels.

Ernst Grohne (1932, 43–57) holds that these cups may have originated in ancient libation rites or drinking/feasting ceremonies. During the medieval and modern periods they are known to have been used by small groups or brotherhoods, where arms were also linked while drinking. This practice might be related to the intertwined handles found on many modern examples (Grohne 1932, Plate 7; Haberey 1953, 82). The brotherhood aspect is most clearly exemplified by a Roman first-century cup from Colchester, Essex, England where a human arm is rising from the foot of one cup to grasp the centre of that next to it (Haberey 1953, 81; Kaye 1914, 175–176).

In the high Middle Ages these cups were also linked to Trinitarian symbolism, where Christ is depicted as triple-headed (Grohne 1932, 32–43; Lexow 1958, 77–99). This may also relate to much older customs, for triplicates of different forms (i.e. triads, triple-headed deities, figures and items) are known from previous periods in many areas (Arnold 1999, 77; Green 1992, 114–116, 149–150, 214–216; 1998; Grohne 1932, 44–48; Kirfel 1948; Lexow 1958, 55–77; Tresidder 2004, 475). On the golden horns of Gallehus in South Jutland in Denmark there is a naked man with three heads (Müller and Jiriczek 1897, 155, fig. 99), and in *Skírnismál* ('Sayings of Skírnir', verse 31 – Holm-Olsen, 1985) Skírnir meets a three-headed troll. Another Scandinavian example is the statue depicting Thor, Odin and Frey in Old Uppsala, Sweden (Davidson 1982, 74).

The Celtic pantheon is formed by several triadic groups, for example, the three craftsmen gods (Green 1992, 214). The Celtic goddess, and the later Christian Saint Brigid, controlled three spheres: healing, crafts and poetry; while the statue of Thor, Odin and Frey may be an example of a Norse trinity working together. Interestingly, the very act of brewing is built on the triple foundation of nature's own ingredients, the craftsmanship of brewing and the wisdom and healing gained from the drink. These three different spheres also reflect the life-cycles and abilities of alcohol in mythology (Davidson 1988, 39; 1993, 112; 1998, 35–37, 67, 88, 135; Green 1989, 170; 1992, 50–51, 214; Tresidder 2004, 78, 475). Within the framework and customs of ritual feasting, the trinitarian aspects of religion could lead to the construction or materialization of different kinds of tools and objects, such as the triple cups discussed here. Divine trinities, like the Fates, can be linked to the cult of the dead (Green 1992, 95; Tresidder 2004, 178–179), making the presence of these cups in graves even more interesting.

The importance and symbolic role of the number three or multiples of three seems to be found all over the world (Tresidder 2004, 475), but particularly in the Indo-European tradition (Green 1992, 214; Lexow 1958, 55; Mallory and Adams 1997, 577–581).

According to Jack Tresidder (2004, 475, 487) three was also the number of harmony for Pythagoras and of completeness (having a beginning, middle and an end) for Aristotle. In general three is the most positive number; representing synthesis, reunion, resolution, creativity, versatility, omniscience, birth and growth. The expression 'third time lucky' is ancient, possibly of Greek origin, and in mythology, folklore and legend heroes or heroines are often granted three wishes or trials (Evensberget and Gundersen 1986, 16; Green 1992, 214–216; Tresidder 2004, 475). There seems to be a common desire to give religious beliefs and sacred actions a threefold form.

Bettina Arnold (1999, 76–78) gives many examples of how multiples of three form the preparations for banquets or feasts, the quantities of food and drink, numbers of guests and length of time for consumption featured in Irish and Welsh literature (see also Gautier 2009). Given the ritual and socio-political significance of drinking in ancient society (Dietler 1990), it would not be surprising to see feasting-goods like the triple cups reflecting a connection to divinity, cosmology and the importance of drinking in a grave or another archaeological context (see also Douglas 1972; Sherratt 1995, 11–12).

The association between the archaeological record and literature is in fact most intriguing. If we go back as early as 550 BC, the Hochdorf chieftain buried in a princely grave in Germany may serve as the first example. The chief had nine drinking horns, nine plates and three serving basins in his chamber grave (Arnold 1999, 77). In southeast Norway, my area of research, the commonest combination of vessels forming possible drinking sets is three. In addition, the triangle is often used as a decorative element on ceramics, and the zigzag, a row of triangles, is the most common decorative element on Norwegian pottery of the first five centuries AD.

Obviously caution is necessary when interpreting artefacts as enigmatic as Norwegian triple cups. Pairs seem to be similarly significant, but in the following pages I will try to show multiples of three had a particular meaning. The Norwegian triple cups pictured in Figure 1a–c are from three different counties in southern Norway. The vessel from Hedrum parsonage in Vestfold is out of context but from a mound in a large cemetery with other rich finds. A second find from Ula in Østfold is a simple cremation, but the third one, from Trålum in Aust-Agder, contains typical feasting equipment with six pottery vessels, caulking resins, bone comb, bone pin, burnt bones and bear claws. It is not easy to find good prehistoric parallels with good contexts, but the high-status grave from Güttingen on the border of Switzerland and Germany (Fingerlin 1964) is dated to the sixth century AD and places the triple cups within a milieu of specialized drinking equipment (spoon sieve, ladle, bronze pan, bronze kettle, glass bowl and bucket are among the finds). Like the Norwegian graves, it was also a part of a pre-Christian burial ground, and the finds are similar to many graves with both imported and locally produced drinking equipment from AD 100–600 in northern Europe (i.e. Lund Hansen 1987). A discovery from Västra Karaby, Scania, Sweden shows that triple cups also appear in settlement contexts (Jeppsson 1996).

Old Norse literature contains many references to multiples of three. These sources are much more recent than the finds discussed above, but they seem to include ideas that are older than the time of writing and might be related to the triple cups. Terje Gansum (1999, 459–461, 467–468) has examined number-magic and concludes that it connects to aspects of cosmology, fate, origin and life and death. I would like to draw attention to myth of the mead of inspiration (*Skaldskaparmál* in Snorri's *Prose Edda*) in which the number three is central:

> The god Kvasir was made from the saliva of the Aesir and Vanir making him the wisest of all.
> Kvasir meets the two dwarves, Fjalar and Galar.
> They kill Kvasir and empty his blood in *three* vessels (a kettle called Odrører and two beakers, Son and Bodn).
> His blood is mixed with water and honey making the mead of inspiration.
> The mead is given to the giant Suttung and his daughter Gunnlød who guard it inside a mountain.
> After passing a trial where he has to do the work of *nine* men for Suttung's brother Bauge, Odin wants a drink of the mead as payment, but Suttung will not allow it.
> Odin sneaks into Gunnlød's lair by crawling through a hole in the mountain in the form of a worm. Once there he sleeps with her for *three* nights.
> After that she allows him *three* drinks of the mead, and he empties all *three* vessels.
> Odin brings the mead to gods and humans by escaping Gunnlød and Suttung in the form of a *bird* (eagle).

I would suggest that these vessels are items of ritual importance and, when used for feasting in either real life or at funerary feasts, they reminded the participants of the strong symbolic connotations of the number three. This symbolism connects both the sacred drink it held but also the divine trinity and the unifying connotations of drinking from integrated cups. In fact triplism may be seen as a sign of totality; in the words of Miranda Green (1989, 170), inspired by Pierre Lambrechts, 'the exaltation of the forces of nature, an expression of extreme potency'.

Bird-shaped Pottery

The next category I wish to investigate is the bird-shaped vessel, of which there are two examples in Norway (Fig. 10.2). The bird from Bjerkreim in Rogaland (Fig. 10.2a) is hollow, with an opening in the forehead and the body decorated with lines imitating feathers. The other bird from Ås østre, Sande in Vestfold (Fig. 10.2b), has a richer decoration of feathers and an opening at the back. Although reconstructed, a narrow channel through the neck indicates that the head has served as a spout. The opening in

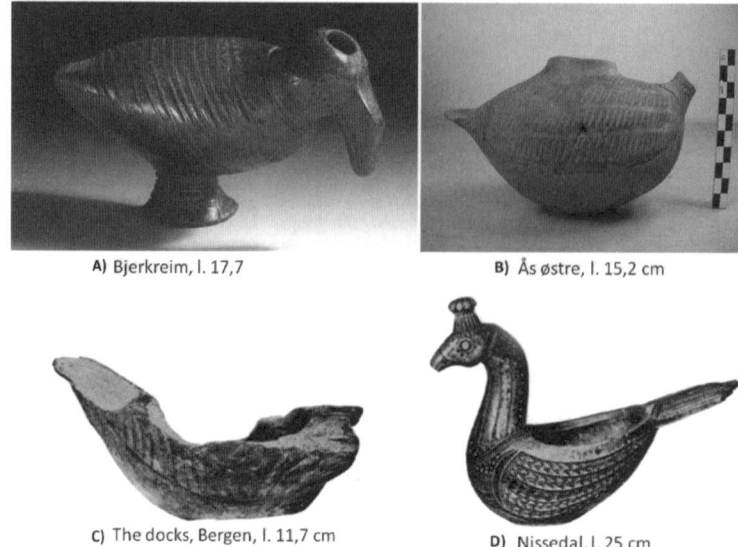

Figure 10.2. Bird-shaped beakers: a) Mus. no. S1413–1422, Bjerkreim, Helleland, Rogaland, Norway, AD 350–450 (photograph, Museum of Archaeology, University of Stavanger); b) Mus. no. C29264, Ås østre, Sande, Vestfold, Norway, AD 300–400 (photograph by the author); c) the docks, Bergen, Norway, fourteenth century (after Gjærder 1975, fig. 255); d) Nissedal, Telemark, Norway, eighteenth century (after Gjærder 1975, fig. 256).

the head seems to be for pouring liquid in both examples, so once again the connection to drinking is unmistakable. Both finds are dated between AD 300–450 (Bøe 1931).

Similar bird-shaped vessels of both metal and ceramics are known from Denmark, Sweden and Holland, and especially from Silesia (Bøe 1931, 131). The use of birds in metalwork, pottery and other drinking vessels goes back to at least the Bronze Age and the Lausitz culture (Kristiansen 1998, 235). Like the triple cups, the birds have parallels in wood (Fig. 10.2 c–d), in Norway dating to the sixteenth/seventeenth centuries. An example with runes (the first part of the futhark) found at the docks in Bergen indicates that the tradition goes back at least to the fourteenth century (Gjærder 1975). A vessel with a handle shaped like a bird, dated to Denmark's early Iron Age, takes the tradition back even further (Visted and Stigum 1951, 127). The fact that they occur in numbers across both geography and time could relate to ancient traditions and mythologies common to many peoples in Europe.

Thus, the vessels may express a basic myth where a life-giving and intoxicating liquid/elixir is brought to humans from the fountain of life by a deity in the form of a bird, like the Odin myth related previously (Hammarstedt 1903, 188–190). Water birds are especially important because of their ability to both fly and swim, thereby being able to help the gods through different elements and reflecting a link between water and air. In the vernacular tradition, birds possess supernatural and prognostic powers, and divine entities like Odin had shamanistic powers, frequently metamorphosing between human and bird form (Green 1992, 43, 69, 85). In Urnfield art (*ca.* 1300–750 BC), ducks are often shown flanking a solar wheel or forming the prow and stern of a boat carrying the sun-disc, while swans often carry wagons with vessels (Green 1989, 89, 203–204; Sprockhoff 1955). Swans are also swimming in the well of life (Urd's well) in Norse mythology (Snorri 2005, *Prose Edda, Gylvaginning* ch. 16). Furthermore the birds at the fountain of life are often featured in art, with the spring represented in the form of a cup or an urn (see Gjærder 1975, fig. 124, 379, 380, 398).

Edvard Hammarstedt (1903, 189–190) claims that the bird in the original myth is supposed to have been a woodpecker, but that the species differs over time. Of essence in this connection is the woodpecker's (especially the green woodpecker's) ability to find and attack bees. In that way it supposedly helped people to find wild honey just as does its relative the greater honeyguide (*Indicator indicator*) in Africa (Short et al. 2003). Honey is, of course, one of nature's sources of sugar, a life-essence for the Greek gods, and possibly the reason why mead is considered a life-giving drink (see also Gjærder 1975, 181, 203–204; Midtun 1921, 138–140).

The use of bird-shaped vessels at ritual meals or feasts would make them very concrete symbols of the myth of the life-giving drink (Gjærder 1975, 180–206). Also this myth seems to lie behind verse 13 in the Old Norse *Hávamál* ('Sayings of the high one') in which:

> A bird of Unmindfulness flutters o'er ale feasts, wiling away men's wits: with the feathers of that fowl I was fettered once in the garths of Gunnlos below.
>
> (Bray 1908)

The ability of birds to fly high in the heavens evokes ideas of freedom and birds could thereby represent the human soul liberated from the body at death. In Old Norse religion, carrion-eaters like ravens and crows are also thought to collect the souls of the dead but at the same time they bring souls back to the world in the form of children. Additionally, they collected wisdom and information from the realm of Mimir in the underworld for Odin, a power also embedded in the life-giving drink (Hammarstedt 1903,193–194). In this connection Mimir's well (containing wisdom and intelligence) could be interpreted as having the same functions as the fountain of life. For Mimir drinks from the well every day, and mead is a kenning for this drink (Snorri, *Prose Edda, Gylvaginning* ch. 15). Singing birds also possessed the powers of enchantment and healing, making them appropriate as thank-offerings (Green 1992, 42, 69, 85, 88,

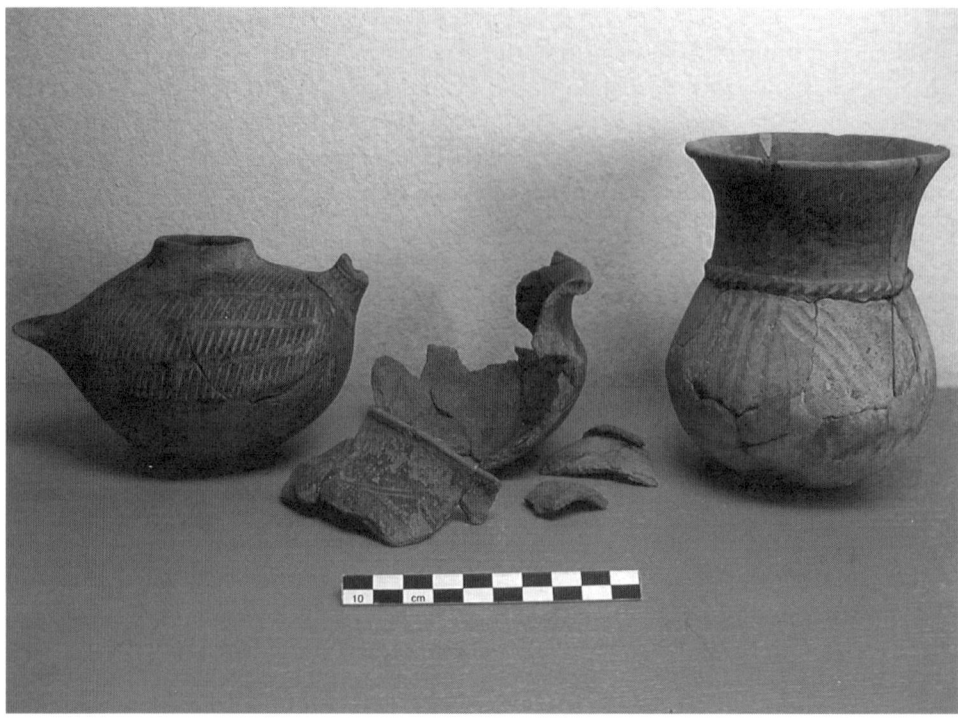

Figure 10.3. Set of three vessels from Ås østre, Sande, Vestfold, Norway, AD 300–400 (photograph by the author).

203–204). The same power can be related to cups in general, but the bird-shaped vessels are key objects when interpreting this symbolism.

Both Norwegian find-contexts with bird-shaped pottery imply that the birds are parts of sets of drinking equipment. The find from Bjerkreim contains many vessels (probably nine or ten) from one or more graves, but they have not been reconstructed. The second from Ås østre forms a set of three vessels (Fig. 10.3), together with caulking resins, iron fragments (perhaps from a sword and nails), a glass bead and burnt bones, again adding to the symbolism of three.

From the evidence presented above it seems possible that bird-shaped cups and also other cups may relate to the myth of the elixir of life, with regenerative powers giving the vessels a particular symbolic quality when used for funerary feasting. The vessels suggest beliefs that the one who drinks from them will gain wisdom but also in regeneration or a new life-cycle for the deceased.

Discussion and Conclusion: the Funerary Feast

The ceramics discussed in this paper are all from graves and are often combined in groups forming sets of drinking equipment, presumably for ritual use. Archaeological finds from the late Hallstatt/early La Tène periods (*ca.* 600–400 BC) and onwards feature the concept of the feast in the world beyond, with grave-goods including provisions and utensils for food and drink (Arnold 2001). When combined with documentary sources (e.g. those dating to *ca.* 300 BC–AD 200 for the Mediterranean and *ca.* AD 600–1200 for Britain and Scandinavia), the socio-political role of drinking and feasting seems to be continuous despite the fact that such a time-frame includes some ideological changes (Arnold 1999; Qviller 2004). The object-types featured in this article should be seen as important symbols in such a wide-reaching concept and indicates that quite distant parallels could be used to interpret these rare cups.

The period with the most elaborate use of feasting equipment in Norway is the first five centuries AD, coinciding with the time when the craft of pottery was at its finest (Bøe 1931). This may be an indication of political struggle, when local chiefs were using feasting equipment competitively, to show off in public so as to claim power. In turbulent periods, strong material symbols relating to cosmology and identity could possibly serve as agents in the contest for power. The cessation of such display in graves might indicate that power relations and prestige items were consolidated (Hedeager 1992, 251). Dispensing large quantities of alcoholic drink to followers is assumed to have been an important element in the political career of a prehistoric leader, with feasting being a recognized institution that had clear socio-political dimensions (Dietler 2001). Praxis theory has proven a valuable tool when trying to reach a deeper understanding of the use of material symbols as opposed to subjects as the only creative agents. Materiality is a non-verbal part of the structuration of praxis (Bourdieu 2000 [1977]). The interrelation of materials and human action is incorporated in habitus – the social praxis through which all agents experience the world (Bourdieu and Wacquant 1993, 37). Presupposing that the agents were acting in a familiar social arena, material objects associated with the institution of feasting would have been recognized by the attendants of the ceremony (Bourdieu and Wacquant 1993, 12, 92–93, 106–107), thereby making such grave-goods important symbols and signifiers of former praxis through experience, memory and movement patterns (Bourdieu 2000 [1977], 72–73, 113; Bourdieu and Wacquant 1993, 112–113). In this way, objects may seem to have an agency of their own, but they are rather the results of social relations made anonymous, reduced to humanized messages from the objects themselves or, in other words, projections for the agents' praxis (Gell 1998, 21; Meskell 2005).

The reason why I have included parallels from different times and places is because I believe that special artefacts, such as the triple-cups and bird-shaped pottery, are key objects to the understanding of prehistoric feasting because of their long-lasting symbolic value. The symbolism embedded in some groups of artefacts is probably the reason why special forms are retained over long periods. They become bearers of tradition and symbolize former praxis and cosmological beliefs. This relates to the double historicity of human society, both bodily dispositions and social-material relations, that Bourdieu (1999, 157–159) describes. The Nordic myth and religion that we are familiar with hardly existed as early as the first centuries AD, but beliefs in triple forms and the bird as an animal that helps and supports seem to be part of much older traditions which can be traced to earlier centuries thanks to archaeological finds and can be illuminated by literary sources such as like Eddic poetry. Following Bourdieu (1996, 61), a symbol is only fully appreciated when more than one agent can relate to it. As seen with the example of the triple cup, the use of this shape has long traditions and probably defined meanings of its own. Similarly, ideas attested in written sources may be much older than the time of their writing.

Symbolism embedded in objects shows how material culture is an integral aspect of society, shaped and produced through human history. Objects might in this way be indicators of qualities of the owner/user (Gell 1998, 13, 108–109). The socio-material world is created through relations between different kinds of beings (e.g. humans, things, animals, plants), thus influencing objects and symbols to become qualities of social life. Through daily repetition, meaning is sustained or reproduced, establishing relations between material culture and human activity (Thomas 1996, 32). The socialization or structuration of material culture is intrinsic to the very constitution of society, stabilizing relations and making the basis of power unquestionable. For Bourdieu (1990, 66–79; 1996, 153; 1999, 144–153), the social and material structures of everyday life are incorporated as dispositions (habitus) in the human body, acting on and perceiving the world. The use and meaning of symbolically loaded artefacts is, then, closely related to the understanding of relations in life and cosmology, working as a reminder for memory and forming human identity through myth, legend and vernacular belief (Altenberg 2003, 36; Odner 2008).

It is my belief that all pottery from graves is related to feasting, but heavily symbolic objects such as triple cups and bird-shaped pottery add a further religious dimension and a wider meaning to the tradition. The strong symbolism embedded in these special pots might also add to the significance of making deals, alliances and agreements while feasting, while the users are reminded of cosmological beliefs and power-relations in society. In general, drinking is a social and collective event, uniting people and communities all over the world. Through material symbols that relate to drinking, the deceased and his/her followers can also use grave rituals as a display of the ability to give feasts in real life, thereby making a statement on the ability as a host and reminding the other participants of their social rank. Thus the funeral ceremony is an important stage for communicating continuity of power structures and sustaining life as it was by the use of strong material symbols.

By way of conclusion, I will return to the use of these cups in British tavern games and Norwegian folk culture. The fact that the same forms appear centuries after the excavated pottery probably indicates that the material symbols are particularly strong. As argued above I believe that the cups originally had an important symbolic function that made those who used them realize a certain history or a religious concept, such as the trinitarian symbolism or the bird as an animal of succour, but it may also refer to a certain social code. As Daniel Miller (2005b, 28) concludes: 'the more humanity reaches toward the conceptualization of the immaterial, the more important the specific form of its materialization'. A core of the original meaning is probably still surviving in the use of these cups in marriage and funeral ceremonies but the meanings might have been renegotiated over time and at some point changed to a more secular or jocular use like the fuddling cup (Monson-Fitzjohn 1927, 42).

References

Altenberg, K. 2003. *Experiencing Landscapes: A Study of Space and Identity in Three Marginal Areas of Medieval Britain and Scandinavia* (Stockholm).
Arnold, B. 1999. '"Drinking the Feast": alcohol and the legitimation of power in Celtic Europe', *Cambridge Archaeological Journal* 9, 71–93.
—— 2001. 'Power drinking in Iron Age Europe', *British Archaeology* 57, 13–19.
Bourdieu, P. 1990. *The Logic of Practice* (Oxford).
—— 1996. *Symbolsk Makt: Artikler i Utvalg* (Oslo).
—— 1999. *Meditasjoner* (Oslo).
—— 2000 [1977]. *Outline of a Theory of Practice* (Cambridge).
——, and Wacquant, L.J.D. 1993. *Den Kritiske Ettertanke: Grunnlag for Samfunnsanalyse* (Oslo).
Bøe, J. 1931. *Jernalderens Keramikk i Norge* (Bergen).
Bray, O. 1908. (ed.) *The Hávamál* (London).
Christie, I.-L. 1986. 'Høne-and-orre. En gruppe fugleformete ølkar. Presentasjon - problemer - spørsmål', *By Og Bygd* 31, 126–166.
Davidson, H.R.E. 1982. *Scandinavian Mythology* (London).
—— 1988. *Myths and Symbols in Pagan Europe: Early Scandinavian and Celtic Religions* (Manchester).
—— 1993. *The Lost Beliefs of Northern Europe* (London).
—— 1998. *Roles of the Northern Goddess* (London).
Dietler, M. 1990. 'Driven by drink: the role of drinking in the political economy and the case of Early Iron Age France', *Journal of Anthropological Archaeology* 9, 352–406.
—— 2001. 'Theorizing the feast: rituals of consumption, commensal politics and power in African contexts', in Dietler, M. and Hayden, B. (eds), *Feasts: Archaeological and Ethnographic Perspectives on Food, Politics and Power* (Washington DC), 65–114.
Douglas, M. 1972. 'Deciphering a meal', *Daedalus* 101, 61–82.
Evensberget, S. and Gundersen, D. 1986. *Bevingede Ord: Nær 12000 Litterære Sitater, Historiske Ytringer, Ordtak og Talemåter, Sentenser og Fyndord* (Oslo).
Fingerlin, G. 1964. *Grab Einer Adligen Frau aus Güttingen* (Freiburg).
Gansum, T. 1999. 'Mythos, logos, ritus: symbolisme og gravskikk i lys av gudediktene i den eldre Edda', in Fuglestvedt, I., Gansum, T. and Opedal, A. (eds) *Et Hus med Mange rom: Vennebok til Bjørn Myhre på 60-årsdagen*. AmS-Rapport 11. (Stavanger), 441–503.
Gautier, A. 2009. 'Hospitality in pre-viking Anglo-Saxon England', *Early Medieval Europe* 17, 23–44.
Gell, A. 1998. *Art and Agency: An Anthropological Theory* (Oxford).
Gjærder, P. 1975. *Norske Drikkekar av Tre* (Bergen).
Glørstad, H. and Hedeager, L. 2009. *Six Essays on the Materiality of Society and Culture* (Lindome).
Green, M.J. 1989. *Symbol and Image in Celtic Religious Art* (London).
—— 1992. *Dictionary of Celtic Myth and Legend* (London).

—— 1998. 'Crossing the boundaries: triple horns and emblematic transference', *European Journal of Archaeology* 1, 219–240.

Grohne, E. 1932. *Die Koppel-, Ring- und Tyllengefässe: ein Betrag zur Typologi und Zweckgeschicht Keramischer Formen* (Bremen).

Haberey, W. 1953. 'Ein Römisches ringgefäss aus Kärlich, Landkreis Koblenz', *Festschrift Römisch-Germanischen Zentralmuseums in Mainz zur Feier seines hundertjährigen Bestehens 1952*. Band 3. (Mainz), 79–82.

Hammarstedt, E. 1903. 'Fågeln med segerstenen, språngörten och lifsämnet', *Meddelanden från Nordiska Museet* 1901, 166–208.

Hedeager, L. 1992. *Iron-Age Societies: From Tribe to State in Northern Europe, 500 BC to AD 700* (Oxford).

Holm-Olsen, L. 1985. (ed.) *Skírnismál* (Skirnesmål), (Oslo).

Jeppsson, A. 1996. 'Boplats och gravar. Karaby 3:1, 4:1, V Karaby socken, RAÄ 39, Stamledning P 36', in Räf, E. (ed.) *Skåne på längden. Sydgasundersökningarna 1983–1985. Arkeologiska Undersökningar* (Lund), 117–166.

Kaye, W. J. 1914. 'Roman and other triple vases', *The Antiquary: A Magazine Devoted to the Study of the Past* 50, 172–177.

Kirfel, W. 1948. *Die dreiköpfige Gottheit: Archæologisch-Ethnologischer Streifzug durch die Ikonographie der Religionen* (Bonn).

Kristiansen, K. 1998. *Europe Before History* (Cambridge).

Lexow, J.H. 1958. 'Trehodete guder og djevler i Norden', *Stavanger Museums Årbok* 67, 55–101.

Lund Hansen, U. 1987. *Römischer Import im Norden: Warenaustausch zwischen dem Römischen Reich und dem freien Germanien während der Kaiserzeit unter besonderer Berücksichtigung Nordeuropas* (København).

Mallory, J.P. and Adams, D.Q. 1997. *Encyclopedia of Indo-European Culture* (London).

Meskell, L. 2005. 'Objects in the mirror appear closer than they are', in Miller, D. (ed.) *Materiality* (Durham, NC), 51–71.

Midtun, G. 1921. 'Drikkekar fra landet i 1600- og 1700-årene', in Vogt, N. (ed.) *Schous Bryggeri: Mindeskrift til Hundredaarsjubilæet 1921* (Kristiania), 126–152.

Miller, D. 2005a. *Materiality* (Durham, NC).

—— 2005b. 'Materiality: An introduction', in Miller, D. (ed.) *Materiality*. (Durham, NC), 1–50.

Monson-Fitzjohn, G.J. 1927. *Drinking Vessels of By-gone Days: From the Neolithic Age to the Georgian Period*, (London).

Müller, S. and Jiriczek, O.L. 1897. *Nordische Altertumskunde: nach Funden und Denkmälern aus Dänemark und Schleswig*. Band II, Eisenzeit, (Strassburg).

Odner, K. 2008. 'Saami sacrifices: materiality and biography of things', in Glørstad, H. and Hedeager, L. (eds) *Materiality. Six Essays on the Materiality of Society and Culture* (Uddevalla), 59–86.

Qviller, B. 2004. *Bottles and Battles: The Rise and Fall of the Dionysian Mode of Cultural Production. A Study in Political Anthropology and Institutions in Greece and Western Europe* (Oslo).

Sherratt, A. 1995. 'Alcohol and its alternatives: symbol and substance in pre-industrial cultures', in Goodman, J., Lovejoy, P.E. and Sherratt, A. (eds) *Consuming Habits: Drugs in History and Anthropology* (London), 11–46.

Short, L., Hancock, J. and Diamond, A.W. 2003. 'Honeyguides', in Perrins, C. (ed.) *The New Encyclopedia of Birds* (Oxford), 656.

Snorri, S. 2005. (trans. Byock, J.L.) *The Prose Edda : Norse Mythology* (London).

Sprockhoff, E. 1955. 'Central European Urnfield Culture and Celtic La Tène: an outline', *Proceedings of the Prehistoric Society* 21, 257–281.

Thomas, J. 1996. *Time, Culture and Identity: An Interpretative Archaeology* (London).

Tilley, C. 2006. *Handbook of Material Culture* (London).

Tresidder, J. 2004. *The Complete Dictionary of Symbols in Myth, Art and Literature* (London).

Veeck, W. 1931. *Die Alamannen in Württemberg* (Berlin).

Visted, K. and Stigum, H. 1951. *Vår Gamle Bondekultur*. Bind 2 (Oslo).

Animals in the Household: Not Just a Foodstuff

Aixa Vidal, Universidad Complutense de Madrid; Instituto Nacional de Antropología y Pensamiento Latinoamericano
and
Ruth Maicas, Museo Arqueológico Nacional, Universidad Autónoma de Madrid

In most societies, talking about food and drink implies talking about animals, but animals have a much wider role in human society than the mere provision of dietary sustenance. When analysing medieval households, Serjeantson (2000) noted the diversity of situations that link animals to humans: they are often companions even if kept for work, sport or food production. In death, their carcasses can be converted into objects, such as bone tools or ornaments, which represent a variety of activities, from technical processing of raw materials to hierarchical symbolism. Meadows (1999) also focused on the role of animals within households, demonstrating that analysis at the domestic level provides a useful context for interpreting archaeological remains.

'Household', however, is a complex concept in archaeological terms and is characterized in various ways (e.g. Alexander 1999, 79; Allison 1999). We define it as a *locus* for indoor social gathering. It is not only the focus of daily subsistence activities, but the social sphere where most interactions take place (Padder 1993). Meaning is given to household spaces through the dynamic relationships between social actors (be they people or animals), the environment and other material elements.

Reconstructing the meanings attached to households in the prehistoric world is a difficult task, as the past functions carried out in this social *locus* would probably have been more diverse than they are today. Animal remains offer an important source of evidence for understanding these activities but, traditionally, studies of faunal remains have been compartmentalized, with animals viewed either as food, raw materials or symbols. Studies of preindustrial societies, however, indicate that human–animal relationships are usually blended, with most activities being integrated in terms of their performance and meaning (Ingold 2002). In this paper we seek to highlight the wide range of roles that animals would have played within prehistoric households, illustrating our argument with examples from the Neolithic to the Late Bronze Age in the Spanish Mediterranean region.

Living with Animals in Prehistoric Spain
The landscape of many areas of the Spanish Mediterranean basin has changed radically

since the later prehistoric period, when the region was more humid. The faunal panorama of later prehistory was, however, similar to today, including a healthy population of game species such as boar, deer and lagomorphs, as well as the domestic horse, which was introduced to Spain in the Chalcolithic period, *ca.* 3200 BC (Pose and Vazquez 2005). Now, as in the past, the area's economy is based on caprines (mainly sheep), together with cattle and pigs. Faunal analyses of archaeological assemblages indicate that dogs and other carnivores were present in low numbers, with birds, microfauna and molluscs also contributing to the region's resource-base (Maicas 2007; Pérez Ripoll 1999). All these animals would have been involved at different levels with their contemporary human societies and their presence within a household, either as living creatures or animal products, would have contributed to its definition in both physical and social terms (Allison 1999).

Of the wide range of activities performed within a household, food processing, storage and consumption are the most widely documented in the archaeological record. However, when discussing food, not only foods should be considered, but the processes and implements involved in cooking and dining should also be examined. For instance, it seems likely that animals played a central role in the process of cooking, particularly by providing bones, fats and dung as a source of fuel: ethnographic studies of herding societies (Miller 1984) have shown that dung is an excellent fuel for heating, cooking and pyrotechnologies. The great advantage of dung is that it burns slowly, which is particularly useful in processing foods that demand long cooking times, such as grains and other high-starch staples of past agricultural populations (Zohary and Hopf 2000). Dung may also be incorporated into clay as a tempering material so that pottery is more porous once fired and, as a consequence, is more resistant to thermal shock (Rye 1981). Unfortunately, organic components disintegrate when the pots are fired, so that evidence for its prehistoric use is only indirect. Better documented is the use of crushed and burnt bone, both as a pottery temper and to infill engraved decoration (Delibes 2008). Recently, it has been suggested that both milk and blood were used in place of water to improve the workability of clays with low plasticity (Vidal forthcoming).

Food storage, of critical importance once settlement became sedentary and a surplus was being produced (Chapman 1991), required not only proper conditions but also appropriate vessels. Some containers made of hide or animal gut could have fulfilled this function, but their short life-span vitiated their efficacy. The shelf-life of containers might be increased by using a combination of ceramic vessels with hide lids. Where it was necessary to generate anaerobic conditions, a sealing or preserving substance could have been used: vinegar and salt were common in Phoenician trade and perhaps earlier, as shown in salty and fermented remains in Neolithic pottery. Regarding animals, fats and honey complemented the range of preserving options available for prehistoric societies (Martín et al. 2005).

Warm animal fats may also have been used to burnish pottery, lithics and bone materials (Edholm and Wilder 2001). The thermal alteration of materials in the domestic

Animals in the Household: Not Just a Foodstuff

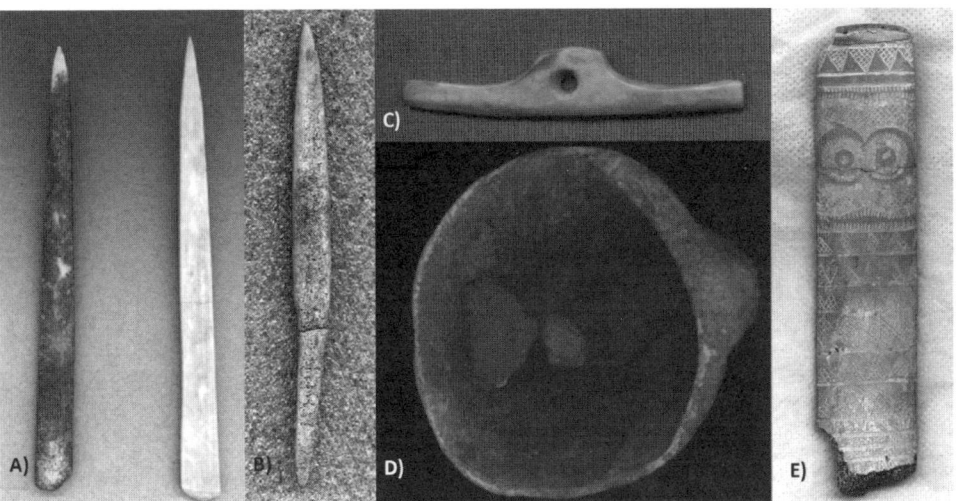

Figure 11.1. Some tools made of animal materials from Almizaraque (Almería): a) pointed tools; b) arrowpoint; c) button; d) shell vessel with ochre; e) oculated idol on rib bone.

fire is another example of a technical process intimately related to cooking; burnt and boiled bones were most probably not discarded but transformed into different tools and artefacts (Speth 2000). The link between bone object manufacturing and culinary processes is also reflected, for instance, in the use of the percussion technique to break bones for the marrow and the resulting flakes subsequently shaped into objects (Sidera 2004). The specific uses of such tools may define separate working areas (LaMota and Schiffer 1999), some of them directly related to feeding practices.

Spoons are, perhaps, the artefacts most directly involved in food processing and consumption, and their presence has been recorded at a large number of sites, in particular those of Neolithic date, along the Mediterranean basin and in northern Europe (see Vidal and Mallía, this volume). Whilst people ate it seems that they may have been entertained by music, which could also be created through animal products: bone flutes were found in L'Or (Martí et al. 2001) and probably in the Spanish southeast (Maicas 2007), whereas whistles and horns of *Charonia nodifera* were identified by Siret (1908) in Los Millares.

Once dinner was finished, bones were not just discarded: in every household there were individuals ready to make good use of them. For dogs they were a source of food and for craftsmen a source of raw materials. Bone tools, daggers and arrow points (Fig. 11.1a, b) have been discovered at many Spanish sites and good examples of long arrow and projectile points come from Almizaraque (Maicas 2007). Personal ornaments have been much discussed elsewhere; in the Spanish south-east, they include a large variety of beads, pendants, buttons and combs made of bone, as well as hide and shell ornaments used by household members of all ages (Fig. 11.1c). For children, bones may have represented fun and entertainment, as is noted among ethnographic societies (Victor and Robert-Lamblin 1989), with some artefacts serving as toys, like the set of phalanges from the Spanish south-east (Maicas 2007).

Due to their hardness, shell tools and objects are frequent finds, even in inland locations (Maicas and Vidal 2010). Glycymerys, Cerastoderma and Acanthocardia valves served as potters' tools, another craft usually performed inside the household living area. The use of shells is exemplified in the decoration of the famous cardial pottery and also in some scrapers or burnishers that, from the position of abrasive traces and their overall size, would have been unsuitable as personal ornaments. Curved bone paddles, specially adapted to pottery-making, were recorded in Andalusia (Meneses 1994). Different organic and inorganic remains such as lipids, varnishes and pigments were identified in the interior of valves from Chalcolithic south-eastern sites (Fig. 11.1d). In some cases, the remains preserved were identified as bitumen (Siret and Siret 1890), probably used as mastic to haft lithic tools or to mend valuable pottery (Connan 1999). The presence of this substance inside the valves suggests that shells were sometimes used as short-term containers.

Soft animal tissue and by-products are rare in the record, but were probably as useful as bone and shell. Animal hides must have been used for a variety of functions in the domestic sphere: clothes, ropes, lids for containers and whole containers, though seldom preserved, were probably made of hide or animal gut. A similar situation is recorded for tendons and hair, although the evidence comes from outside the area of

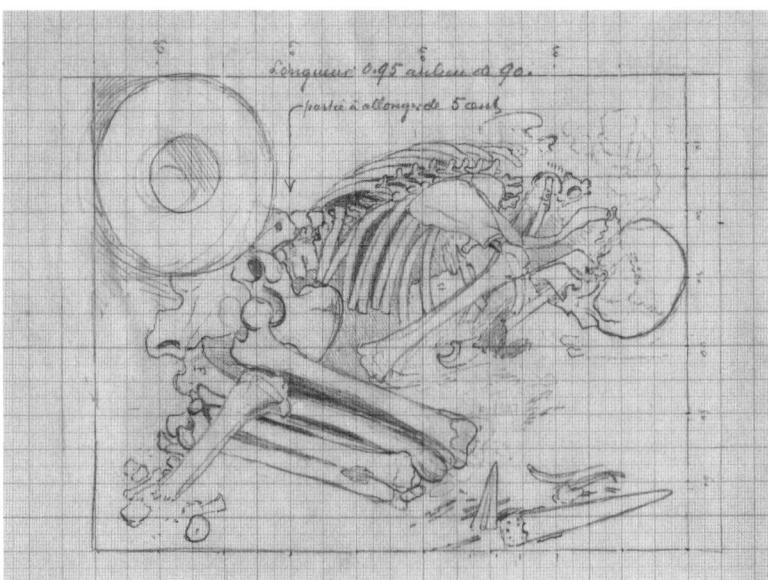

Figure 11.2. Siret's drawing of the Cista de Mina Ibéria (Almería). Argaric burial with an important offering of meat (bovid tibia).

Animals in the Household: Not Just a Foodstuff

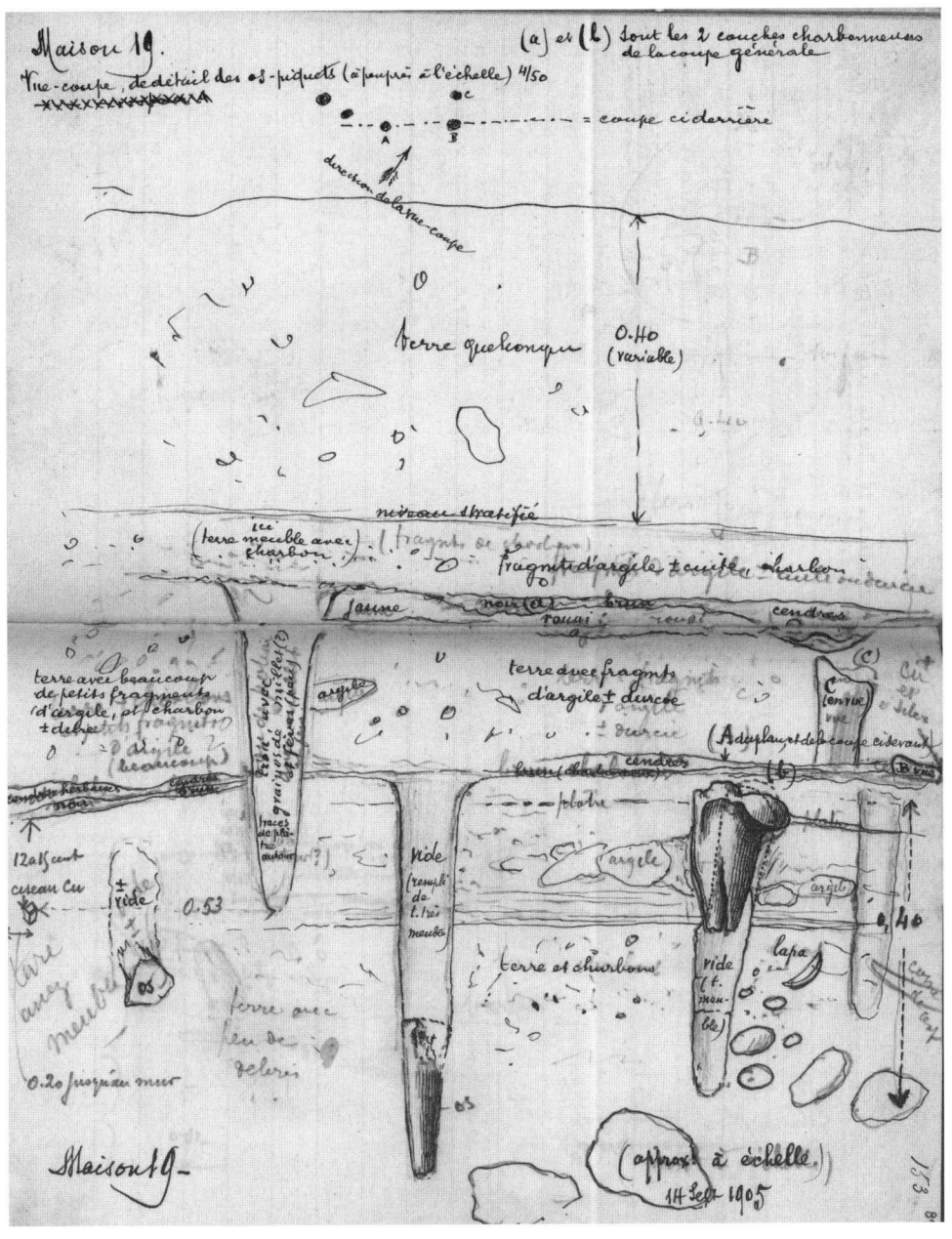

Figure 11.3. Bone structure recorded in Siret's notebooks.

study (Sager 2008). Regarding wool, its use has been postulated for Spanish sites since the Final Neolithic (Pérez Ripoll 1999). So far, there is no direct evidence of feathers as clothing or ornaments, but their use can be assumed on the basis of the feather-like headdresses depicted in post-Palaeolithic Levantine rock art (Roldán et al. 2005).

Analysis of rock art and pigment reservoirs has verified that animal fats, urine and blood were all used in cave paintings (García et al. 2004). It seems likely that these substances were also used in body-paints: thus, animals served as an interface between the functional and aesthetic. Leaving aside the vertebrates, colourants can be obtained from cuttlefish, *Murex* sp., or insects such as *Kermes*, documented in this area for protohistoric societies (Roquero 2002).

As is the case in many societies today, animals were presumably crucial for medical treatments. The use of milk for feeding infants and elderly people, as well as a means of producing long-lasting foods such as cheese — evident in the cheese-maker sherds found in some south-eastern sites (Enguix 1981) — is commonly considered one of the advantages of the by-product revolution (Sherratt 1981). Milk and animal fats can be used as lotions for skin diseases; certainly these were widely appreciated in Roman times and perhaps earlier, as interpreted in the painted bottle from El Tarajal (Almagro Gorbea 1974). Toads, snakes and other poisonous species could have been exploited for their venom; besides their postulated importance as hallucinogens (Lewis-Williams and Pearce 2005), they may have relieved pains and repelled insects. Even nowadays, cobwebs are applied to cuts and bruises to stop bleeding (Luna 2005).

Beyond providing humans with medical remedies, animals may also have offered spiritual sustenance or helped to order society by acting as trophies or identity markers: for instance the deer canines, carnivores' teeth and boar tusks in many sites of the Spanish south-east may have been used to signify an individual or group's hunting rights over particular taxa (Chapman 1991). Certainly the intrinsic value of deer canines was so high by the Final Neolithic that shell reproductions of them were common grave-goods (Maicas and Vidal 2010). Human burials, such as that from Almería (Fig. 11.2), have also been found to contain animal bones, which probably acted as offerings that reflected the status of the deceased.

The symbolic use of animals is visible in portable artefacts like zoomorphic vessels (e.g. Cuesta de la Sabina, Gor), or clay appliqués in Chalcolithic Almería sites that are thought to represent deities and/or acting as offerings (Siret 1908). Almería is also noteworthy because of some peculiar bone structures identified by Siret (1908) where bone pegs formed an oval enclosure around a large number of clay crescents (Fig. 11.3). Although the function of this structure is still unclear, it may have related to household activities (Maicas 2007).

Also related to the symbolic aspect of animals is the world of idols: the Spanish south-east and the Levant are well known for bone figurines, especially the oculated idols (Fig. 1e) manufactured on long bones from different taxa (ovicaprids, bovids, suids and equids), with a complex decoration and iconographic system (Maicas 2007).

Conclusion

The direct and indirect use of faunal resources provided prehistoric societies with a fundamental source of shelter, fuel, containers, processing utensils, ornaments, ritual implements and even companionship. The relative importance of animals in the economic and social life of different groups must have varied over time and cultural context, but the nature of the relationship between animals and humans was certainly always close if not familiar.

Our aim here was to discuss one of the many possible pictures of human life in the prehistoric Spanish Mediterranean basin, specifically regarding animal participation in everyday life. We believe that the non-edible uses for animals and their related by-products were profoundly embedded into routine household organization, almost as much as they were valued as a nutritional resource.

References

Alexander, R. 1999. 'Mesoamerican house lots and archaeological site structure: Problems of inference in Yaxcaba, Yucatan, Mexico, 1750–1847', in Allison, P. (ed.) *The Archaeology of Household Activities* (London), 78–100.

Allison, P. 1999. 'Introduction', in Allison, P. (ed.) *The Archaeology of Household Activities* (London), 1–18.

Almagro Gorbea, M. 1974. 'Un nuevo recipiente pintado del Bronce Antiguo almeriense', *Trabajos de Prehistoria* 31, 317–27.

Chapman, R. 1991. *La Formación de las Sociedades Complejas* (Barcelona).

Connan, J. 1999. 'Use and trade of bitumen in antiquity and prehistory: molecular archaeology reveals secrets of past civilizations', *Philosophical Transactions of the Royal Society of London* 354, 33–50.

Delibes, G. 2008. 'La colección de vasos campaniformes', in Zulueta, P. and Escobar, I. (eds) *El Tesoro Arqueológico de la Hispanic Society of America* (Alcalá de Henares), 270–285.

Edholm, S. and Wilder, T. 2001. *Buckskin: The Ancient Art of Braintanning* (Boonville).

Enguix, R. 1981. 'Queseras halladas en los yacimientos del Bronce valenciano', *Archivo de Prehistoria Levantina* 16, 251–80.

García, P., Domingo, I., Roldán, C., Verdasco, C., Ferrero, J., Jardón, P. and Bernabeu, J. 2004. 'Aproximación al uso de la material colorante en la Cova de l'Or', *Recerques del Museu d'Alcoi* 13, 35–52.

Ingold, T. 2002. *The Perception of the Environment. Essays on Livelihood, Dwelling and Skill* (London).

LaMotta, V. and Schiffer, M. 1999. 'Formation processes of house floor assemblages', in Allison, P. (ed.) *The Archaeology of Household Activities* (London), 20–42.

Lewis-Williams, D. and D. Pearce. 2005. *Inside the Neolithic Mind* (London).

Luna, R. 2005. *Dorland Diccionario Enciclopédico Ilustrado de Medicina* (Barcelona).

Maicas, R. 2007. *Industria ósea y funcionalidad: Neolítico y Calcolítico en la Cuenca de Vera.* (Madrid).

—— and Vidal, A. 2010. 'More than food: beads and shell tools in Late Prehistory in the Spanish Southeast', in *Munibe,* Suplemento 31, Proceedings of the 2nd Archaeomalacology Working Group Meeting (Santander), 168–175.

Martí, B., Arias-Gago, A., Martínez R. and Juan-Cabanilles J. 2001. 'Los tubos de hueso de la Cova de L'Or (Beniarrés, Alicante). Instrumentos musicales en el Neolítico Antiguo de la Península Ibérica', *Trabajos de Prehistoria*, 58(2), 41–67.

Martín, A., Martín, J., Villalba, M., Juan-Tresserras, J. 2005. 'Can l'Oliaire (Berga, Barcelona), un asentamiento neolítico en el umbral del IV milenio con residuos de sal y de productos lácteos', *III Congreso del Neolítico en la Península Ibérica* (Santander), 175–186.

Meadows, K. 1999. 'The appetites of households in early Roman Britain', in Allison, P. (ed.) *The Archaeology of Household Activities* (London, Routledge), 101–20.

Meneses, M. 1994. 'Útiles de hueso del Neolítico final del sur de la Península Ibérica empleados en Alfarería: placas curvas, biseles, placas y apuntados', *Trabajos de Prehistoria* 51, 143–156.

Miller, N. 1984. 'The use of dung as fuel: an ethnographic example and an archaeological application', *Paléorient* 10(2), 71–79.

Padder, E. 1993. 'Spatiality and social change: domestic space in Mexico and the United States', *American Ethnologist* 20(1), 114–37.

Pose Nieto, H. and Vázquez Varela, J. 2005. 'Nuevos datos y perspectivas sobre la domesticación del caballo: los caballos criados en régimen de libertad en Galicia, Noroeste de España', *Munibe* 57, 487–493.

Pérez Ripoll, M. 1999. 'La explotación ganadera durante el III milenio a. C. en la Península Ibérica', *II Congrés del Neolític a la Península Ibèrica, Saguntum Extra 2*, (Valencia), 95–103.

Roldán, C., Murcia-Mascarós, S., Ferrero, J., Villaverde, V., Martínez, R., Guillem, P. and López, E. 2005. 'Análisis *in situ* de pinturas rupestres levantinas mediante EDXRF', *Proceedings of the VI Congreso Ibérico de Arqueometría* (Girona), 203–210.

Roquero, A. 2002. 'Tintorería en la Antigua Roma. Una tecnología al servicio de las artes suntuarias', in González Tascón, I. (ed.), *Artifex. Ingeniería Romana en España* (Madrid), 51–55.

Rye, O. 1981. *Pottery Technology: Principles and Reconstruction* (Washington).

Sagger, R. 2008. *Hair Today, Gone Tomorrow: The Degradation and Conservation of Archeological Hair Fibers*. Unpublished MA Thesis. Texas A&M University.

Serjeantson, D. 2000. 'Good to eat *and* good to think with: classifying animals from complex sites', in Rowley-Conwy, P. (ed.) *Animal Bones, Human Societies*, 179–189 (Oxford).

Sherratt, A. 1981. 'Plough and pastoralism: aspects of the secondary products revolution', in Hodder, I., Isaac, G. and Hammond, N. (eds) *Pattern of the Past: Studies in Honour of David Clarke* (Cambridge), 261–305.

Sidera, I. 2004. 'L'Industrie de l'Os Préhistorique: Matières et techniques', *Cahier XI* (Paris).

Siret, H. and Siret, L. 1890: *Las Primeras Edades del Metal en el Sudeste de España* (Barcelona).

Siret, L. 1995 [1908]. *Religiones neolíticas de Iberia*. Colección Siret de Arqueología 2. (Almería).

Speth, J. 2000. 'Boiling *vs.* baking and roasting: a taphonomic approach to the recognition of cooking techniques in small mammals', in Rowley-Conwy, P. (ed.) *Animal Bones, Human Societies* (Oxford), 89–105.

Victor, P. and Robert-Lamblin, J. 1989. *La Civilisation du Phoque: Jeux, Gestes et Techniques des Eskimo d'Ammassalik* (Paris).

Vidal, A. Forthcoming. 'Identificación de agregados líquidos en pastas cerámicas', *Proceedings of the II Congreso Internacional de Arqueología Experimental*.

Zohary, D. and Hopf, M. 2000. *Domestication of Plants in the Old World* (Oxford).

Feasting and the State in Uruk Mesopotamia

Jessica L. Whalen, University of Edinburgh

One theme predominates in fourth- and third-millennium iconography from Mesopotamia: the feast, which is depicted in standardized and highly formulaic ways (Boese 1971, Plates 1–38; Pinnock 1994, 24; Schmandt-Besserat 2001, 397; Pollock 2003, 22). The appearance of glyptic representations of feasting is coincident with the first city-states of the Uruk period (4000–3100 BC) and the associated shifts in social stratification, settlement patterning, agriculture and architecture. Key features of Mesopotamian city-states – e.g. the extent of centralization, the role of private rural industries, mass-produced ceramics and precious worked items – are still debated (Adams 1981, 125; Beale 1978, 503; Millard 1988, 52; Chazan and Lehner 1990, 30). This is perhaps because the evidence has traditionally been subject to 'top-down' interpretations which tend to view any socio-economic shift as the product of large, all-encompassing central agencies.

This paper adopts a 'bottom up' approach and considers whether the shifts in Uruk-period society might have resulted from individual agency at a community level, whereby feasting was used to accumulate influence and extract labour outside of large-scale complexes. Evidence is collated from a number of Uruk-period sites, the location of the most significant being shown in Figure 12.1.

Anthroplogical and Archaeological Approaches to Feasting

Anthropological literature has attempted to categorize different types of feasts, constructing typologies of feasting behaviour. Particular attention has been given to differentiating between 'celebratory' feasts, those held for the purpose of social bonding, and 'competitive' feasts, which serve to create and maintain social distance (Dietler 1990, 1996, 2001; Dietler and Hayden 2001a, 2001b; Hayden 1996, 2001, 2003). Researchers have also defined an intermediate category, named 'patron-role' (Dietler 1996, 96–97) or 'redistribution' feasts (Hayden 1996, 129), whereby individuals elicit the labour of others in exchange for hosting a feast when the work is finished. As such, individuals with the capital to host feasts are able to extract labour directly from the community, thereby increasing both tangible wealth and social prestige. The key here is that hosting need not be restricted to the uppermost social classes; it is possible amongst any segment that finds itself able to consolidate capital to spend on large-scale provision of food and drink. In this way it is possible for any individual within a community to create debts and accumulate influence or political control.

Within the archaeological record, feasting may be detected through the presence of special foods and feasting items, or by identifying emulation, a feature of 'competitive'

Feasting and the State in Uruk Mesopotamia

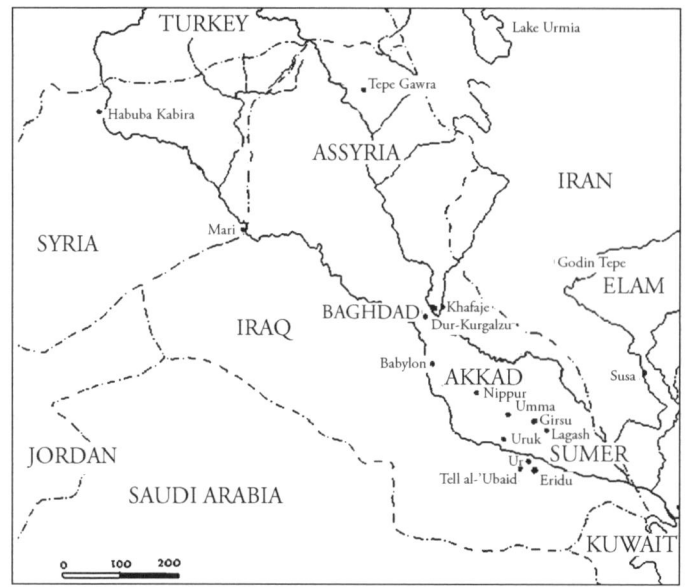

Figure 12.1. Map showing sites mentioned in the text.

feasting. Hayden (1996, 137) has outlined a number of potential traits for identifying feasting in archaeological contexts:

1) abundant resource bases capable of providing surpluses;
2) special foods used for feasting;
3) special vessels used for serving feasting food;
4) the use of prestige items that food surpluses can be converted into;
5) the occurrence of special grounds or structures where feasting events could be held;
6) the occurrence of 'Triple A' individuals having more wealth and influence than others in the community.

This paper will focus on the evidence from categories two and five. By considering the presence of special foods and the occurrence of special places, it is hoped that it will be possible to identify Hayden's (1996, 132) 'Triple A' personalities, those 'ambitious, aggressive accumulators/aggrandizers/acquirers' who manage to extract labour and capital from others in return for participation or other, less tangible social rewards.

Detecting Special Foods (Alcohol Consumption) in the Uruk Period

Archaeologically, the detection of 'special foods' has been most successful with alcohol. For instance, chemical analysis was undertaken on ceramic samples from a 50-litre jar from fourth millennium contexts at Godin Tepe, a large fortified site along Zagros trade routes, and identified the presence of calcium oxalate (McGovern 2003, 160), a compound associated with beer-making (Homan 2004, 86). The jar featured a small hole at its sidewall, suggesting beer was drunk from the jar via long straws or tubes, as is seen on early sealing images. McGovern notes similar jars with spouts or holes at their rims 'extending up to Mari on the Euphrates, across Turkey, and out into the Aegean Sea to the Cycladic island of Naxos' (McGovern 2003, 160). A four-spouted krater was found within early third millennium BC levels at Karataş in Lycia, modern Turkey (Mellink 1969), and it is possible that ring-vases, which appear at early third-millennium sites along the western Anatolian coast, were similarly used for beer drinking (Whalen forthcoming). Long straws as beer-drinking paraphernalia (see Homan 2004, 86) have been recovered in precious materials, such as in gold from the Royal Cemetery of Ur (Katz and Voigt 1986, fig. 11) or of metal from Hittite levels at Alaca Höyük (Koşay and Akok 1951, Plate LV). Prestigious prototypes indicate this was an activity enjoyed by élites at the time; yet this should not colour our perception that beer was consumed only by élite groups: the most common forms of straws or drinking tubes were likely of reeds, which are unlikely to have survived.

Beer production is evidenced in Uruk Mesopotamia. At Lagash (modern Tell al-Hiba) the remains of an ancient brewery were discovered, complete with a large oven, 'tanks' or vats used for mixing, and dough mixed with herbs (Hansen 1980–83, 426–30). At Girsu (modern Telloh), temple accounts record that barley was issued to brewers and mention the quality of beer received in return (Powell 1994, 93). Dating from the twenty-fourth century BC, they comprise one of the earliest direct references to beer and indicate it was an important enough commodity to have warranted the issue of barley for its production, as well as to have been purposely extracted by city authority.

In terms of wine consumption, the most compelling evidence comes from Early and Late Period V at Godin Tepe (3500–2900 BC), contemporary with the Late Uruk period. Tartaric acid was detected chemically in jars whose tapering, piriform shape suggest developing insight into wine product storage (McGovern and Michel 1996, 61; Badler 1996, 49–50). It is possible that these jars were transported to the south; piriform jars have been excavated from Late Uruk contexts at several sites, including Uruk, Nippur, and Girsu, Susa in south-western Iran, and at Habuba Kabira and Tepe Sialk along northern Late Uruk trade routes (McGovern 2003, 162). Chemical analysis has also been undertaken on Uruk-period ceramics from Susa, Girsu and Uruk; samples from droop-spouted jugs all indicated the presence of resinated wine (ibid., 162). The form of the jugs, in particular their curved spouts, rendered them less than ideal as vessels for wine transport (ibid., 161); however, their use as commensal items is evident from glyptics of the Early Dynastic period (see Fig. 12.2). Droop-spouted vessels continue to be found in assemblages throughout the succeeding Jemdet Nasr (3100–2900 BC) and Early Dynastic (2900–2350 BC) periods, suggesting the culture of the Late Uruk had become familiar with wine to the extent that its use was increasingly accessible to, and imitated by, larger population segments (Adams and Nissen 1972, 100–03).

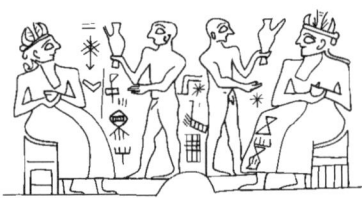

Figure 12.2. Perforated plaque from Nippur featuring droop-spouted jar (after Boese 1971, Plate 18, 8).

Evidence for Special Places

Public plazas appear as early as temples, and are generally associated with public buildings. Uruk's Eanna Precinct, which is flanked by three temples (Red, C and D), features a large elevated terrace with ample space for hosting special events made all the more dramatic by the plaza's lofty location (Nissen 1970; Lloyd 1978, 51). Similar open plazas are found at most major Uruk temples but over the course of the period appear to shift away from open design towards increased construction of protective enclosures for guarding the sanctuaries (Forest 1999, 89).

At Tepe Gawra, we may see a connection between the plaza and large-scale food preparation and consumption. Here, the earliest Ubaid constructions (5000–3500 BC) feature a public plaza flanked by three 'obviously religious buildings' (Lloyd 1978, 75). During the Early Uruk period, a secular building was added to the complex and food-preparation and serving rooms – indicated by the presence of hearths, serving vessels, large bowls, cooking pots and possibly a bread oven – were built around one of the temple's courtyards (Rothman 2002, 93–94). The area was clearly a place for public gatherings (ibid., 107) and, although it could have functioned simply as a market place, its connection with food preparation tempts the conclusion that it could have hosted large-scale consumption events.

Restricted access to special foods is often reflective of wider socio-political changes. At Godin Tepe, Badler (1996) has noted wine drinking changes from open practice to private activity between Early and Late period V, coincident with the Late Uruk period. During Early Period V (3500–3100 BC), most wine jars are found in a large room off of a central courtyard. No doors connect the room to the courtyard, but rather two windows at waist height. Associated with the windows were a large cache of around 2000 slingballs, piled as if they were part of a distribution system effected through this room (Badler 1996, 52). Inside the room were large immovable jars, their interiors stained red (ibid., 53), while a large open-mouthed jar contained beer residue (Michel et al. 1992, 1993). If this room functioned as distribution centre, it seems wine and beer were some of the items given out. Yet in succeeding Late Period V (3100–2900 BC) wine drinking is detected only in small, private rooms (Badler 1996, 53). Wine jars recovered from a 'luxury residence' – a room with curtained wall and fine plastered floor – had chipped necks, indicating they were opened and their contents consumed within the room (ibid., 53). Badler has noted that the change in context wherein wine is found – from open, distributed item to private and restricted – mirrors socio-economic shifts of the settlement. In Late V, Late Uruk influence declines at Godin Tepe in favour of Transcaucasian influence: a reduction in Uruk tablets, cylinder seals and sealings is noted at the same time that Transcaucasian pottery comes to represent up to one-third of the assemblage (ibid., 55). To Badler, this suggests the supply of wine became increasingly restricted within the hands of a small group of élite, who rose to prominence with the decline of Mesopotamian centralized systems. Of course, these two groups could use wine in different ways. But it is also likely that wine, a luxury item then as now, was a salient indicator of status, and access to this symbol was controlled not only by economics but also ideological factors. Wine drinking, an emblem of élite participation, became increasingly controlled as the socio-political character of the settlement changed.

Feasting within Domestic Settings

Domestic architecture of the Uruk period offers insight into how food preparation may be used to obtain social influence outside large institutions. Uruk houses were typically closely connected and arranged around inner courtyards. At Habuba Kabira South, houses of the period were commonly positioned around large halls, many of which contained inner courtyards, fireplaces and small attached chambers, interpreted as for hosting communal events (Kohlmeyer 1996, 97). These structures were accessible only by careful navigation of corridors and alleys between houses, suggesting that they were only used by those familiar with the twists and turns of the domestic areas of the town. Over time, and in particular during the following Early Dynastic period, houses increased in scale and elaboration, while central spaces became a standard feature of domestic architecture (Lebeau 1996, 132). Such trends suggest gathering was important amongst urban non-élite populations, and that as households gained in prestige, residents chose to devote more space to gatherings. This connection between gathering and private wealth may well indicate a positive trend, in which gathering promoted, and perhaps was cause for, social mobility, and perhaps was a viable means by which individuals were able to consolidate social and economic capital.

House construction provides a means by which feasting may have been used amongst populations outside central complexes. Building a house in the Uruk period was complicated; the presence of professional builders is poorly evidenced even in the third millennium (Kolínski 1996, 137). This means that for the average Uruk family, house construction would have relied upon neighbours. Labour may have been procured through systems of reciprocal obligation, or the provision of incentive. This seems the very situation anthropologists Dietler (1996, 94) and Hayden (1996, 128–9) detail in their description of the 'work-party' feast, whereby individuals are rewarded for their participation in collective building activities through the provision of food.

Ceramics of the Uruk period, while lacking in the aestheticism generally associated with feasting contexts, demonstrate how communal imbibement may reflect socio-economic developments. As opposed to the painted wares and rich decoration of the preceding Ubaid period, 90 per cent of Early Uruk wares are unpainted (Adams and Nissen 1972, 100), and by the Late Uruk, simple and crudely made bevelled-rim bowls make up at least 50 per cent of assemblages at many sites (Chazan and Lehner 1990, 26). Previous interpretations of these bowls as a ration item issued by central complexes (Nissen 1970, 137; Johnson 1973, 132) are contradicted by their similarly-proportioned distribution in both rural and urban areas (Adams 1981, 125), suggesting use not only by central institutions, but also on a local level. If these bowls are taken merely as an indication of food production and consumption, their distribution seems to indicate more appropriately the presence of gathering, and thereby within rural and non-élite contexts, at large-scale religious and secular institutions. Their proposed use in ritual presentation (Beale 1978, 305) corresponds well with depictions of simple, hand-held bowls in feasting processions on the Uruk vase (ibid., 307), while interpretation as bread mould (Chazan and Lehner 1990; Millard 1988, 52) could denote gathering amongst rural and non-centralized domestic groups. As feasting is an effective means to draw people together and induce political support, perhaps these bowls, with their widespread presence in all contexts of the period, suggests social mobility was present amongst the middle and lower classes, and was achieved or expressed, as anthropologists suggest, through food.

Conclusion

Feasting was pervasive in Late Uruk culture, within non-élite populations as much as élite, in domestic as well as public spheres. The increasing abundance of jars with perforated rims, long straws, 'wine storage' jars and droop-spouted jugs suggests a number of individuals were familiar with, and utilized, special foods, including archaeochemically-detected beer and wine. Mass-produced vessels may, by their similar distribution at large and small sites, show the ubiquity of this consumption, and perhaps gathering at community level. Architecture of the period demonstrates the opportunity for collective imbibement within both public and private spheres, and amongst non-élite populations.

Commensal politics provides insight into Uruk social organization. As anthropological theory details, the provision and display of foodstuffs is a tangible expression of access differentiation, and is a process begun early amongst all societal levels, for the purposes of labour elicitation, wealth redistribution, and accumulation of social capital. Patron-role and redistribution feasts, so labelled by Dietler (1996) and Hayden (1996), are a means by which influence and wealth could be accumulated amongst non-élite populations. Competitive feasting was likely practised amongst these populations just as amongst the élite. In the following Early Dynastic period, feasting themes in artistic reliefs and continual elaboration of feasting-related paraphernalia suggest these activities took on an even more common role in the construction and maintenance of social hierarchies; these processes were begun in the Early Uruk period and we must look for their impact during the rise of the first states. Thus the role of food and drink in societies may not only illuminate the daily lives of previously ignored populations, but help to reconstruct economic practices and provide a more comprehensive and realistic view of societal structure altogether.

References

Adams, R.M. 1981. *Heartland of Cities* (London).
—— and Nissen, H.J. 1972. *The Uruk Countryside: The Natural Setting of Urban Societies* (London).
Badler, V.R. 1996. 'The archaeological evidence for winemaking, distribution, and consumption at Proto-Historic Godin Tepe, Iran', in McGovern, P.E., Fleming, S.J. and Katz, S.H. (eds) *The Origins and Ancient History of Wine* (Amsterdam), 45–56.
Beale, T.W. 1978. 'Bevelled rim bowls and their implications for change and economic organization in the later fourth millennium BC', *Journal of Near Eastern Studies* 37(4), 289–313.
Boese, J. 1971. *Altmesopotamische Weihplatten*. Walter de Gruyter (Berlin).
Chazan, M. and Lehner, M. 1990. 'An ancient analogy: pot baked bread in ancient Egypt and Mesopotamia', *Paléorient* 16(2), 21–35.
Dietler, M. 1990. 'Driven by drink: the role of drinking in the political economy and the case of early Iron Age France', *Journal of Anthropological Archaeology* 9, 366–70.
—— 1996. 'Feasts and commensal politics in the political economy: food, power and status in Prehistoric Europe', in Weissner, P. and Schiefenhövel, W. (eds), *Food and the Status Quest: An Interdisciplinary Perspective* (Oxford), 87–125.
—— 2001. 'Theorizing the feast: rituals of consumption, commensal politics, and power in African contexts', in Dietler, M. and Hayden, B. (eds) *Feasts: Archaeological and Ethnographic Perspectives on Food, Politics, and Power* (London), 65–114.
—— and Hayden, B. 2001a. *Feasts: Archaeological and Ethnographic Perspectives on Food, Politics and Power* (Washington DC).
—— and Hayden, B. 2001b. 'Digesting the feast: good to eat, good to drink, good to think', in Dietler, M. and Hayden, B. (eds), *Feasts: Archaeological and Ethnographic Perspectives on Food, Politics and Power* (Washington DC), 1–20.
Forest, J.D. 1999. *Les premiers temples de Mésopotamie: 4e et 3e millénaires*. (Oxford, BAR Series 765).
Hansen, D.P. 1980–83. 'Lagaš', in Weidner, E. and von Soden, W. (eds) *Reallexikon der Assyriologie und Vorderasiatischen Archäologie* 6 (Oxford, BAR Series 132), 426–30.
Hayden, B. 1996. 'Feasting in prehistoric and traditional societies', in Weissner, P. and Schiefenhövel, W. (eds), *Food and the Status Quest: An Interdisciplinary Perspective* (Oxford), 127–147.
—— 2001. 'Fabulous feasts: a prolegomenon to the importance of feasting', in Dietler, M. and Hayden, B. (eds), *Feasts: Archaeological and Ethnographic Perspectives on Food, Politics, and Power* (London), 23–64.
—— 2003. 'Were luxury foods the first domesticates? Ethnoarchaeological perspectives from Southeast Asia', *World Archaeology* 34(3), 458–69.
Homan, M.M. 2004. 'Beer and its drinkers: an ancient Near Eastern love story', *Near Eastern Archaeology* 67(2), 84–95.
Johnson, G.A. 1973. *Local Exchange and Early State Development in Southwestern Iran* (Ann Arbor).
Katz, S.H. and Voigt, M.M. 1986. 'Bread and beer: the early use of cereals in the human diet', *Expedition* 28, 23–34.
Kohlmeyer, K. 1996. 'Houses in Habuba Kabira South: spatial organisation and planning of Late Uruk residential architecture', in Veenhof, K.R. (ed.), *Houses and Households in Ancient Mesopotamia: Papers read at the 40th Recontre Assyriologique Internationale, July 5–8, 1993, Leiden* (Istanbul), 89–104.

Kolínski, R. 1996. 'Building a house in third millennium northern Mesopotamia: when vision collides with reality', in Veenhof, K.R. (ed.) *Houses and Households in Ancient Mesopotamia: Papers Read at the 40th Rencontre Assyriologique Internationale, July 5–8, 1993, Leiden* (Istanbul), 137–44.

Koşay, H. Z. and Akok, M. 1951. *Alacahöyük kazisi 1937–1939. Türk Tarih Kurumu Basimevi* (Ankara).

Lebeau, M. 1996. 'Les maisons de Melebiya. Approche fonctionelle de l'habitat privé au IIIe millénaire av. notre ère en Haute Mésopotamie', in Veenhof, K.R. (ed.) *Houses and Households in Ancient Mesopotamia: Papers Read at the 40th Rencontre Assyriologique Internationale, July 5–8, 1993, Leiden* (Istanbul), 129–36.

Lloyd, S. 1978. *The Archaeology of Mesopotamia* (London).

McGovern, P.E. 2003. *Ancient Wine: The Scientific Search for the Origins of Viniculture* (Princeton).

—— and Michel, R.H. 1996. 'The analytical and archaeological challenge of detecting ancient wine: two case studies from the Ancient Near East', in McGovern, P.E., Fleming, S.J. and S.H. Katz (eds) *The Origins and Ancient History of Wine* (Amsterdam), 57–66.

Mellink, M. 1969. A four-spouted krater from Karataş. *Anadolu* 13, 69–76.

Michel, R.H., McGovern, P.E. and Badler, V.R. 1992. 'The chemical confirmation of beer from protohistoric Mesopotamia', *Nature* 360, 24.

——, McGovern, P.E. and Badler, V.R. 1993. 'The first wine and beer: chemical detection of ancient fermented beverages', *Analytical Chemistry* 65, 408A–413A.

Millard, A.R. 1988. 'The bevel rim bowls: their purpose and significance', *Iraq* 50, 49–57.

Nissen, H. 1970. 'Grabung in den Qadraten K/L XII in Uruk-Warka', *Baghader Mitteilungen* 5, 101–191.

Pinnock, F. 1994. 'Considerations on the "banquet theme" in the figurative art of Mesopotamia and Syria', in Milano, L. (ed.) *Drinking in Ancient Societies: History and Culture of Drinks in the Ancient Near East, Vol VI. Papers of a Symposium Held in Rome, May 17–19 1990* (Padova), 15–26.

Pollock, S. 2003. 'Feasts, funerals and fast food in early Mesopotamian states', in Bray, T.L. (ed.) *The Archaeology and Politics of Food and Feasting in Early States and Empires* (New York), 17–38.

Powell, M.A. 1994. 'Metron ariston: measure as a tool for studying beer in ancient Mesopotamia', in Milano, L. (ed.) *Drinking in Ancient Societies: History and Culture of Drinks in the Ancient Near East* (Padova), 91–119.

Rothman, M.S. 2002. *Tepe Gawra: The Evolution of a Small Prehistoric Center in Northern Iraq* (Philadelphia).

Schmandt-Besserat, D. 2001. 'Feasting in the ancient Near East', in Dietler, M. and Hayden, B. (eds) *Feasts: Archaeological and Ethnographic Perspectives on Food, Politics and Power* (Washington DC), 391–403.

Whalen, J. forthcoming. PhD dissertation, 'Wine, feasting and prestige networks in Early Bronze Age central and western Anatolia'. University of Edinburgh.

Cleaning Grain and Making Beer: Analysis of a Third- to Fourth-Century AD Archaeobotanical Assemblage from Bottisham, Cambridge

Kate Parks, University of Leicester

The case study presented here forms part of a wider study into Iron Age and Roman arable practice in the east of England that seeks to identify which crops were grown in these periods and how they were cultivated as well as determining how cereals were processed and stored.

This paper focuses on the archaeobotanical assemblage from a single site: Tunbridge Lane in Bottisham, Cambridgeshire. The site was excavated by Archaeological Solutions in 2006–7 and has been interpreted as an outlying area of a farmstead or small settlement dating to the third to fourth centuries AD (McConnell et al. 2008). Features included two substantial third-century 'corndriers' in an area enclosed by a curvilinear gully (Fig. 13.1). The excavation strategy included widespread bulk-sampling; this study is based on the 136 samples taken from phased contexts (the 'corndriers' and various open contexts). Archaeobotanical data, methodology and in-depth discussion are presented in the site archaeobotanical report (Nicholson 2008).

The Crops

Poor preservation meant that almost half of grains could not be identified as to species. Spelt wheat is the best represented crop (31 per cent), with barley also present in significant quantities (18 per cent). Spelt wheat glume bases and barley rachis fragments are also present. A single barley-rich sample containing no spelt wheat indicates that barley was cultivated in its own right as well as growing within the spelt crop. Small quantities of bread wheat were present, along with even smaller amounts of oats (possibly wild) and pulses. These are thought to have grown incidentally in the spelt and barley crops. Other weeds are scarce in the assemblage, accounting for just 8 per cent of all identifications.

Cultivation Practice

Cultivation practice was elicited using autecological analysis of the weed assemblage of the spelt crop (after Van der Veen 1992) to assess soil fertility (nitrogen content) and acidity, supported by identification of weed perennation to assess the level of soil disturbance. *Bromus* sp. accounted for 25 per cent of the weed assemblage; analysis was carried out both including and excluding (as presented here) this species but this was

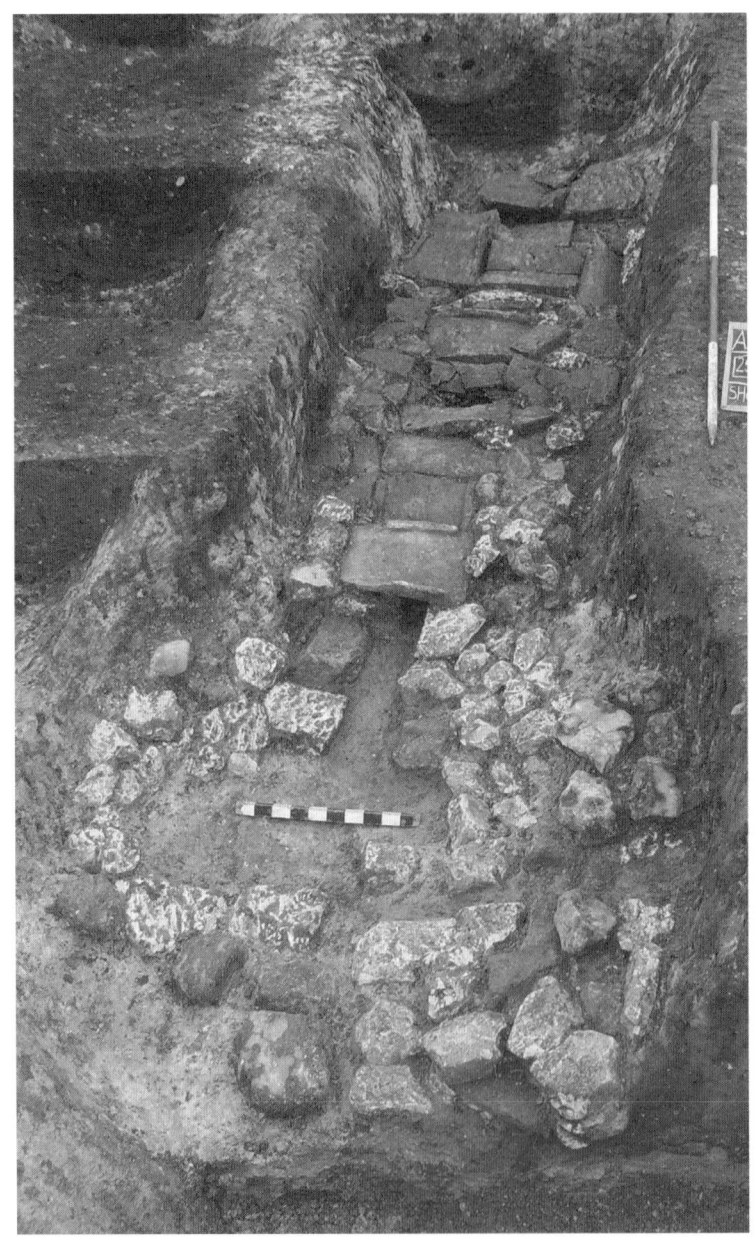

Figure 13.1. The larger 'corndrier' (photograph by Archaeological Solutions).

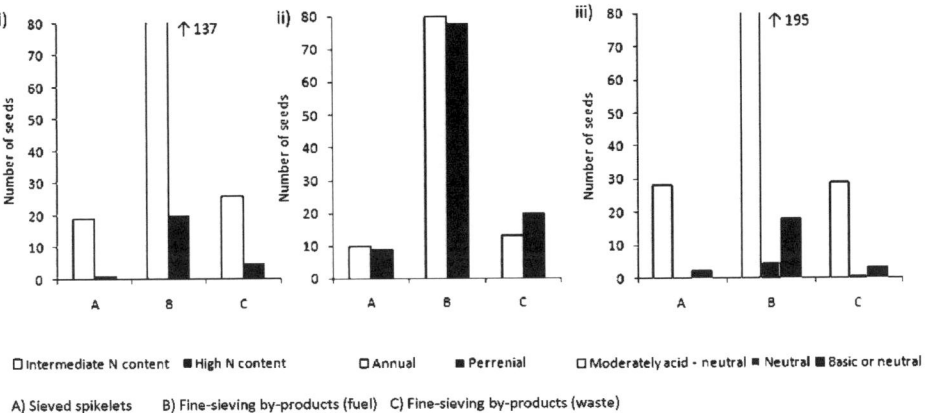

Figure 13.2. i) Weed autecological indication of soil nitrogen content; ii) weed perennation; iii) weed autecological indication of soil acidity.

found not to affect the interpretation of cultivation practice. To counter the effects of crop processing on the composition of weed assemblage, it was subdivided into groups of like crop processing derivation (A, B and C, see Fig. 13. 2) prior to analysis.

The weed species give no indication of nitrogen-depleted soils (Fig. 13.2a), but also very little evidence of the nitrogen-rich soils which would suggest efforts to improve soil fertility (e.g. manuring, fallowing or tillage/aeration). Low levels of disturbance, i.e. infrequent tillage, are also suggested by the high proportion of perennial weed species (Fig. 13.2b). The dominance of species of moderately acidic soils (Fig. 13.2c) is surprising in this area of chalk bedrock and basic modern soils. Combined with the evidence for intermediate soil nitrogen content, this suggests a degree of soil exhaustion. Together, this evidence points to an extensive cultivation regime, in which crop yields were probably ensured by the planting of large areas, rather than by the investment of labour or resources to improve soil fertility (Van der Veen 1992, 148).

Cleaning Grain and Making Beer

The sequence of crop processing employed at the site (Fig. 13.3) was identified through the calculation of ratios of major crop components (after Van der Veen 1992, 82–84; 2007; Van der Veen and Jones 2006) and the ratio of germinated to ungerminated grain (after Van der Veen 1989).

Crop Processing and Storage

The early stages of crop processing were evidenced only by very occasional rachis and straw fragments. Twenty-six assemblages representing the by-products of the later stages of crop processing contained relatively sparse plant macrofossils and probably

Cleaning Grain and Making Beer

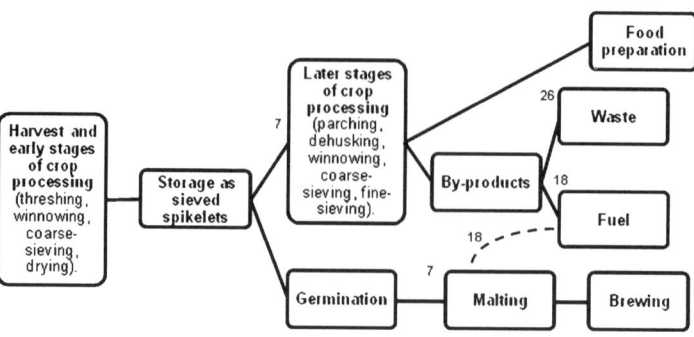

Figure 13.3. Crop processing sequence (numbers indicate number of samples representing each stage).

accumulated gradually (cf. Van der Veen and Jones 2006; Van der Veen 2007). This suggests that these later crop processing stages were carried out piecemeal, as grain was required for food preparation, and that spelt grain was initially stored in spikelet form (i.e. while still contained in its glumes). The scarcity of weed seeds, particularly those of small size, in all samples suggests that the spikelets had been sieved before storage. Seven sparse samples interpreted as spikelets are thought to have been accidentally burnt during parching to facilitate dehusking. Their sparseness suggests that this was not carried out *en masse*, and so supports the conjecture that grain was stored prior to the later stages of processing.

Evidence for Roman grain storage practice in this region is scarce, but assemblages from a late-third/fourth century granary destroyed by fire at Great Holt's Farm, Boreham, Essex, indicate the storage of clean grain (and pulses), separated by species (Murphy and De Moulins 2002). Storage of spelt wheat in spikelet form had been normal practice in the region in the Iron Age and has the advantage of reducing susceptibility to spoilage (ibid.).

Malting
A further seven samples interpreted as spelt spikelets contained high proportions of germinated grain (up to 70 per cent), so are thought to have been accidentally burnt during malting. Malting in spikelet form has previously been recognized at Roman Mucking (Van der Veen 1988). Eighteen samples with dense plant macrofossils represent a mixture of crop processing by-products burnt as fuel and germinated grain, attesting the use of such by-products to fuel the malting process. All of these malting-related samples were from contexts associated with or close to the two 'corndriers', indicating

that these were used for malting. Large-scale malting has also been identified at other Roman sites in the region, including Stebbing Green, Essex (Murphy 1999), and Beck Row, Mildenhall, Suffolk (Fryer 2004). The use of crop processing by-products to fuel the process was also identified at both of these sites.

A further 18 samples of dense plant macrofossils representing spelt processing by-products are also thought to have been used as fuel (cf. Van der Veen and Jones 2006; Van der Veen 2007). These may represent fuel used for other (unidentified) processes, or fuel used for malting on occasions when no grain was accidentally burnt, though their spatial association with the malting ovens was less clear than that of the samples mentioned above.

Conclusions

This study has identified an extensive cultivation regime, with low investment of labour/resources in crop cultivation. It has also identified a low input of labour/resources after the harvest, necessitating the storage of crops in spikelet form and an increase in the day-to-day workload of those responsible for food preparation. This could indicate low availability or small-scale organization of labour (cf. Stevens 2003). However, in this case it seems likely that resources were more profitably invested in malting and the production of beer. This practice is attested by the presence of two substantial malting ovens as well as by the interpretation of archaeobotanical samples as representing accidentally burnt malt and fuel for the malting process. Malting on this scale is consistent with the production of beer for sale in a market economy. This suggests that the occupants of the site at Tunbridge Lane were participating in such an economy, and were investing their labour and resources in the way that most increased the economic value of their crop (cf. Van der Veen and O'Connor 1998).

References

Fryer, V. 2004. 'Charred plant macrofossils and other remains', in Bales, E. (ed.) *A Roman Maltings at Beck Row, Mildenhall, Suffolk* (East Anglian Archaeology Occasional Paper 20), 49–54.

McConnell, D., Pole, C., Woolhouse, T. and Sparrow, P. 2008. *Land South of Tunbridge Lane, Bottisham, Cambridgeshire, Areas 1 & 2: Archaeological Excavation Interim Report* (Archaeological Solutions Unpublished Report 3036).

Murphy, P. 1999. 'Charred plant remains and molluscs from Roman contexts', in Bedwin, O. and Bedwin, M. (eds.) *A Roman Malt House. Excavations at Stebbing Green, Essex, 1998* (East Anglian Archaeology Occasional Paper 6), 19–21.

—— and de Moulins, D. 2002. *Review of Plant Macrofossils from Archaeological Sites in the East of England and East and West Midlands*. Unpublished draft 12/2002, English Heritage.

Nicholson, K. 2008. *Archaeobotanical Samples from Tunbridge Lane, Bottisham (AS1011)*. Unpublished report prepared for Archaeological Solutions Ltd.

Stevens, C.J. 2003. 'An investigation of agricultural consumption and production: models for prehistoric and Roman Britain', *Environmental Archaeology* 8, 61–76.

Van der Veen, M., 1988 *Carbonized Grain from a Roman Corn-drier at Mucking, Essex* (Ancient Monuments Laboratory Report, Old Series, 3834).

—— 1989. 'Charred grain assemblages from Roman-period corn driers in Britain', *Archaeological Journal* 146, 302–319.

—— 1992. *Crop Husbandry Regimes: An Archaeobotanical Study of Farming in Northern England, 1000 BC – AD 500* (Sheffield).

—— 2007. 'Formation processes of desiccated and carbonised plant remains – the identification of routine practice', *Journal of Archaeological Science* 34, 968–990.

—— and Jones, G. 2006. 'A re-analysis of agricultural production and consumption: implications for understanding the British Iron Age', *Vegetation History and Archaeobotany* 15, 217–228.

—— and O'Connor, T. 1998. 'The expansion of agricultural production in late Iron Age and Roman Britain', in Bayley, J. (ed.), *Science in Archaeology: An Agenda for the Future* (London), 127–143.

The Fauna of the Neolithic Lakeside Settlement of Dispilio, Greek Macedonia

Eleni K. Samartzidou, Aristotle University, Thessaloniki

This short paper focuses on the animal remains recovered from the first lakeside settlement to be excavated in Greece: the site of Dispilio in western Macedonia (prefecture of Kastoria), which lies on the south shore of the lake of Kastoria (Fig. 14.1). Ceramic typologies suggest that the site was occupied sporadically from the Middle Neolithic up to historical times but radiocarbon dates suggest that the most intensive occupation occurred in the Middle and Late Neolithic periods (Fakorellis and Maniatis 2002, 289–293; Sofronidou 2008, 14–20; unpublished radiocarbon dates of Laboratory Dimokritos, Greece).

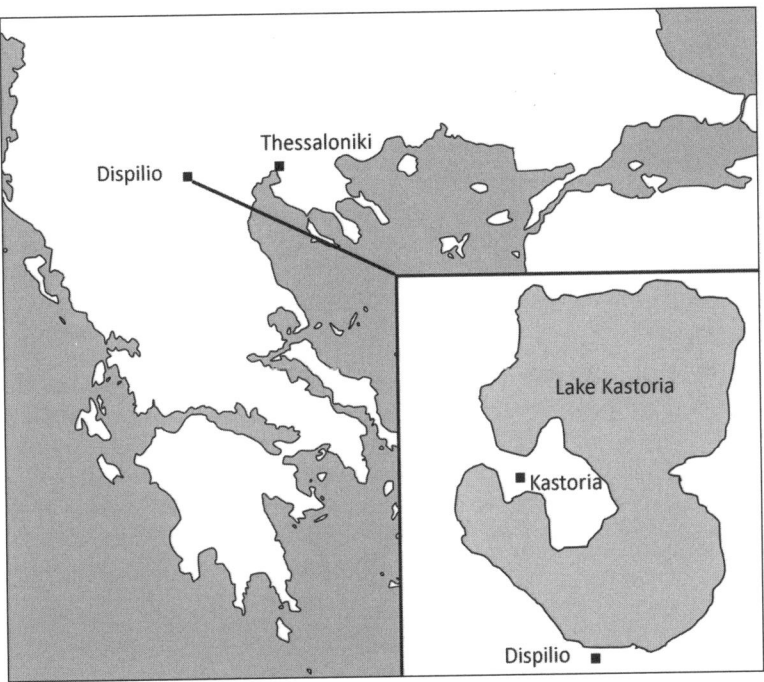

Figure 14.1. Map of western and central Macedonia showing the site of Dispilio.

The Site of Dispilio

At present the extent of the settlement at Dispilio is unknown but research has focused on the site of 'Nisi', a low mound beside the lake shore where undisturbed archaeological deposits have been recovered. Nisi covers *ca.* 17000 m^2 (1.7 ha) and, to date, an area of *ca.* 5250 m^2 (0.525 ha) has been excavated, revealing a number of occupation levels. At a depth of 1.60–2.00m, Phases V and VI are the oldest and date to the Middle and Late Neolithic. Occupation in this period consisted exclusively of a 'lake type' settlement, where houses were positioned over the water. Phases III and IV (depth: 0.80–1.60m) also date to the Middle and Late Neolithic but correspond to a period of 'amphibious type' settlement, where houses were either over the water or beside it, depending on fluctuations in the level of the lake itself. Phases I and II (depth: 0.45–0.80m) were exclusively terrestrial, with houses constructed on dry land, and are dated to Late Neolithic. Above the depth of 0.45m is a surface layer which contains mixed ceramics dating from Neolithic and Bronze Age to historical times. No significant architectural remains were found in this layer, although a few postholes and minor constructions were noted for the Bronze Age, and a stone wall and enclosure were dated to the historical period (Karkanas 2002, 295–302; Sofronidou 2008, 9–25; Hourmouziadi and Giagoulis 2002, 37–74). The natural surface has not been reached in any trench yet. The site is under excavation almost every year.

Results: Preliminary Notes on the Faunal Assemblage of Dispilio

Excavations from 1992 to 2002 have yielded a considerable number (74,190 fragments) of animal bones deriving from the surface layer and phases I–IV. The remains were collected from the whole excavated area and, although sieving was not carried out systematically, recovery was as thorough as possible. The fragments identified to date are shown in Figure 14.1.

Taxa Representation

There are slight inter-period variations in taxa representation – for instance, from the earlier to later phases there is a gradual increase in the representation of wild species – but all phases of the site are dominated by domestic animals. Generally, sheep (*Ovis aries*) are the most abundant, followed by pig (*Sus scrofa domesticus*), cattle (*Bos taurus*), goat (*Capra hircus*) and dog (*Canis familiaris*). The single bone of a domestic cat (*Felis catus*) comes from a disturbed layer. Of the 31 identified equid specimens, most (n=19) come from the surface layer, which is consistent with the traditional belief that horses were introduced to the area during the Bronze Age (Benecke 2006, 93). However some of the bones come from the Neolithic layers and further research is needed in order to determine whether these specimens are intrusive or represent very early imports of this species.

Among the wild taxa, red deer (*Cervus elaphus*) and roe deer (*Capreolus capreolus*) predominate, while the wild boar (*Sus scrofa scrofa*) and the hare (*Lepus capensis*) follow.

The Fauna of the Neolithic Lakeside Settlement of Dispilio

Species	NISP
Human (Homo sapien)	22
Domestic Mammals	
Sheep (Ovis aries)	2320
Goat (Capra hircu)	171
Ovis aries/Capra hircus	4675
Pig (Sus scrofa domesticus)	1783
Cattle (Bos tarus)	644
Dog (Canis familiaris)	423
Cat (Felis catus)	1
Horse (Equus caballus)	31
Wild Mammals	
Aurochs (Bos primagenius)	6
Red deer (Cervus elaphus)	115
Roe deer (Capreolus capreolus)	88
Cervidae	3
Wild boar (Sus scrofa scrofa)	45
Fox (Vulpes vulpes)	11
Brown bear (Ursus arctos)	3
Badger (Meles meles)	5
Marten (Martes foina)	1
Otter (Lutra lutra)	4
Hare (Lepus capensis)	84
Red squirrel (Sciurus vulgaris)	2
Hedgehog (Erinaceous europeaus)	10
Mustelidae	5
Indeteminate Mammals	
Canidae	14
Carnivora	16
Bos/Cervus	16
Ovis/Capra/Cervus	119
Large Mammal	121
Medium Mammal	1838
Rodentia/Insectivora	11
Birds	215
Reptiles and Amphibians	
Tortoise (Testudo spp.)	412
Bufo spp.	2
Rana spp.	2

Figure 14.2. Composition of the identified assemblage from Dispilio in terms of NISP (Number of Identified Specimens).

The least common species, many of which were probably not systematically preferred prey or accidental prey or species that have intruded in the assemblage, are: aurochs (*Bos primigenius*), red fox (*Vulpes vulpes*), brown bear (*Ursus arctos*), badger (*Meles meles*), otter (*Lutra lutra*), marten (*Martes foina*), squirrel (*Sciurus vulgaris*), and hedgehog (*Erinaceus europaeus*). Some bones of Rodentia/Insectivora were also recorded but could not be identified to species level. Bones of frog (Ranidae) and toad (Bufonidae) were also identified. Tortoise (Testudo) bones are fairly well represented in the assemblage, although many of these specimens could be intrusive. It is noteworthy that birds are a systematically targeted game group, although their remains have not, as yet, been analysed in detail.

Exploitation of the Main Domesticates

Throughout Dispilio's occupation, domestic animal husbandry appears to have centred upon food production. Figure 14.2 shows the age-profiles for Dispilio's sheep/goat population, compared with Payne's (1973) model for 'meat production'. Dispilio's caprines exhibit a slightly older average age of death and it would seem that the site's inhabitants were managing their animals for a mixed meat–milk–wool production, though meat was probably the primary goal. Sheep size seems to have increased in later phases, while goat size remains stable. Ageing data suggests that cattle were also raised for meat and milk; there is no pathological evidence to indicate that they were used for traction. From earlier to later phases there is a gradual decrease in the overall size of cattle but pig size remained stable throughout all the periods. As with the other domestic taxa, pigs were maintained primarily for their meat but presumably also as a valuable source of fat.

Spatial Patterning and Carcass Processing

In all occupation levels, discarded body parts seem to have originated mostly from human consumption events rather than from slaughter, skin processing or tool-manufacture. Certainly cattle appear to have been slaughtered outside the excavated area, since very few mandibles from this taxon have been recovered. Skeletal representation for pigs and sheep/goats is more uniform across the site, perhaps suggesting that these smaller animals could be butchered and consumed within the domestic setting. In the case of wild animals, particularly the larger species such as the aurochs, deer and wild boar, it would seem that preliminary butchery took place away from the settlement, probably at the kill-sites, with only selected body parts being brought back to Dispilio. For instance, the assemblage excavated to date contains high frequencies of foot bones (metapodia and phalanges) – obviously attached to hides – and meat-bearing elements but very few cranial fragments have been identified.

The percentages of cut marks (recorded according to Binford 1981) are extremely low in all the occupation levels, but particularly in the later phases. This is probably due to the absence of butchery waste but could equally be explained if the lithic

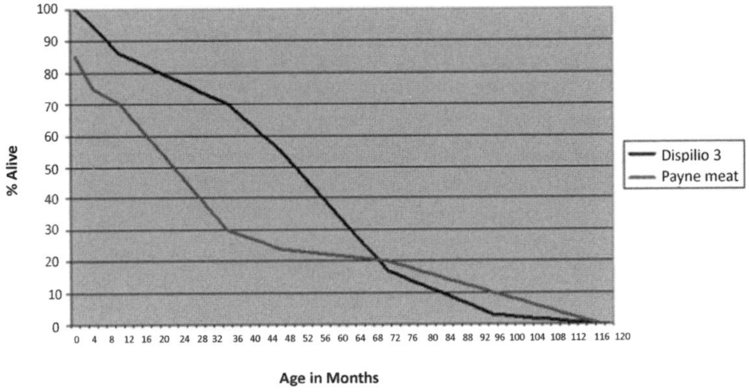

Figure 14.3. Ageing data for Dispilio sheep/goats shown against Payne's (1973) 'meat' model.

butchery tool left little trace on the bones. Dismembering marks were observed most often on sheep/goat bones, less commonly on cattle and pigs. Cattle bones, particularly those belonging to mature individuals, were more frequently fragmented for marrow extraction (according to Binford 1981, 171–177, figs. 4: 52–55), while sheep/goat and pig bones show less evidence of this form of processing. Filleting marks are concentrated in body parts with high nutritional value and they are found not only on the bones of the main domesticates but also dogs, which seem to have been consumed sporadically.

Discussion and Conclusion

Whilst analysis of the site's rich faunal remains has only just begun, it is clear that the results for the lakeside settlement of Dispilio are very similar in nature to those of the toumbas (tell sites) and horizontally extending settlements of the same period in Greece.

In common with published zooarchaeological assemblages from Neolithic Greece, the animal bone material from Dispilio indicates that domestic animals comprise almost 90 per cent of the assemblage, with sheep/goats being particularly well represented, followed by pigs and domestic cattle. Age-at-death patterns for sheep/goat, cattle and pigs indicate that their breeding focused on meat production and, in the case of caprines and cattle, dairying. As with other sites in the Peloponnese and Macedonia, wild mammals approach 8–10 per cent of the total assemblage, with deer species, wild boar and hare being the most numerous (Trantalidou 1996). Consequently, although Dispilio is a unique archaeological site, it does not seems to have been singular in terms of its patterns of animal exploitation: the animal breeding and hunting practices that took place here were comparable to those that took place elsewhere in Neolithic Greece.

References

Benecke, N. 2006. 'On the beginnings of horse husbandry in the southern Balkan Peninsula – the horse bones from Kirklareli-Kanligeçit (Turkish Thrace)', in Mashkour, M. (ed.) *Equids in Time and Space: Essays in Honour of Véra Eisenmann* (Oxford), 92–100.

Binford, L.R. 1981. *Bones, Ancient Men and Modern Myths* (New York).

Fakorellis, G. and Maniatis, G. 2002. 'Apotelesmata chronologisis deigmaton me ti methodo tou 14C', in Hourmouziadis, G.H. (ed.), *Dispilio 7.500 Chronia Meta* (Thessaloniki), 289–294.

Hourmouziadi, A. and Giagkoulis, T. 2002. 'Provlimata kai methodoi proseggisis tou chorou', in Hourmouziadis, G.H. (ed.), *Dispilio 7.500 Chronia Meta* (Thessaloniki), 37–74.

Karkanas, P., 2002. 'I mikromorphologiki meleti ton apotheseon tou Dispiliou', in Hourmouziadis, G.H. (ed.), *Dispilio 7.500 Chronia Meta* (Thessaloniki), 295–305.

Payne, S. 1973. 'Kill-off patterns in sheep and goats: the mandibles from Aşvan Kale', *Anatolian Studies* 23, 281–303.

Sofronidou, M. 2008. 'O proistorikos Limnaios oikismos tou Dispiliou Kastorias: mia proti eisagogi', *Anaskamma* 1, 9–26.

Trantalidou, K. 1996. 'Georgia-Ktinotrofia-Kynigi-Alieia', in Papathanasopoulos, G. A. (ed.) *Neolithikos Politismos stin Ellada* (Athina), 96–101, 231–235.

Eating, Processing and Storing Food in Arid Andean Highlands

Aixa Vidal, Universidad Complutense de Madrid; Instituto Nacional de Antropología y Pensamiento Latinoamericano

The local environment of the southern Andean highlands, with its extreme aridity, great contrast between night and daytime temperatures, seasonal variations and low atmospheric pressure, has always posed a challenge to permanent settlement. Nevertheless, the area has been inhabited since the beginnings of the Holocene, first by hunter-gatherers and later by Formative groups that settled on the plains *ca.* 2400 BP. The Formative period (*ca.* 2400–900 BP) is characterized by a rise in settlement densities and a progressive increase in food production practices, with an important shift from animal herding to agriculture. Towards the end of the period this intensification was accompanied by the development of complex irrigation systems, such as those seen around the site of Bajo del Coypar and the larger neighbouring settlement of Casa Chávez Montículos (Olivera and Vigliani 1999).

The site of Casa Chávez Montículos (hereafter CChM) is located in Antofagasta de la Sierra (north-western Argentina; Fig. 15.1) and is typical for the period. It is a tell settlement that was inhabited from *ca.* 2400 to 1300 BP, with a hiatus in occupation between 2000–1700 BP. The occupational hiatus divides the site's chronology into two clear-cut phases: Early (*ca.* 2400–2000 BP) and Late (*ca.* 1700–1300 BP) (Olivera 1997).

At the beginning of the Formative period (*ca.* 2400 BP), CChM consisted of a simple structure with a small number of tells and there is little evidence that the surrounding landscape was extensively used, perhaps with the exception of highlands herding and ritual activity (Olivera et al. 2003). In this early period, camelid consumption was dominant and lithics were oriented towards hunting and food processing activities. About 2000 BP, the site was seemingly abandoned but was reoccupied in *ca.* 1700 BP when new tells were built in the landscape. The original tells were still utilized, but use of the space appears to have become more segregated both inside the site and in the nearby cemetery and agricultural fields. Flint knapping continued but the period also saw the development of agricultural tools such as shovels, pestles and large containers.

Considerable quantities of pottery were recovered from both phases of CChM and this paper will considered these ceramic assemblages to evaluate whether they provide further evidence to explain the lifestyle change at the settlement.

Eating, Processing and Storing Food in Arid Andean Highlands

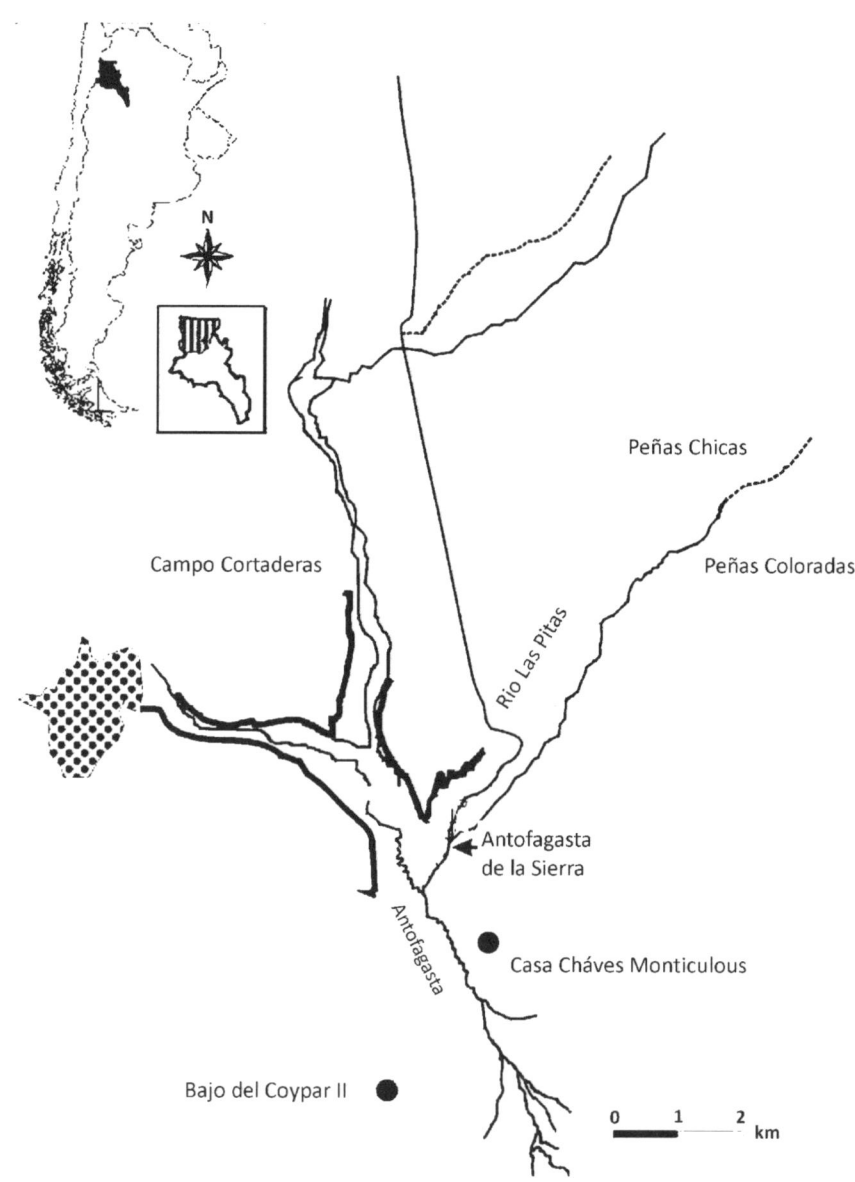

Figure 15.1. Location of Casa Chávez Montículos in Antofagasta de la Sierra (Catamarca, Argentina).

Eating, Processing and Storing Food in Arid Andean Highlands

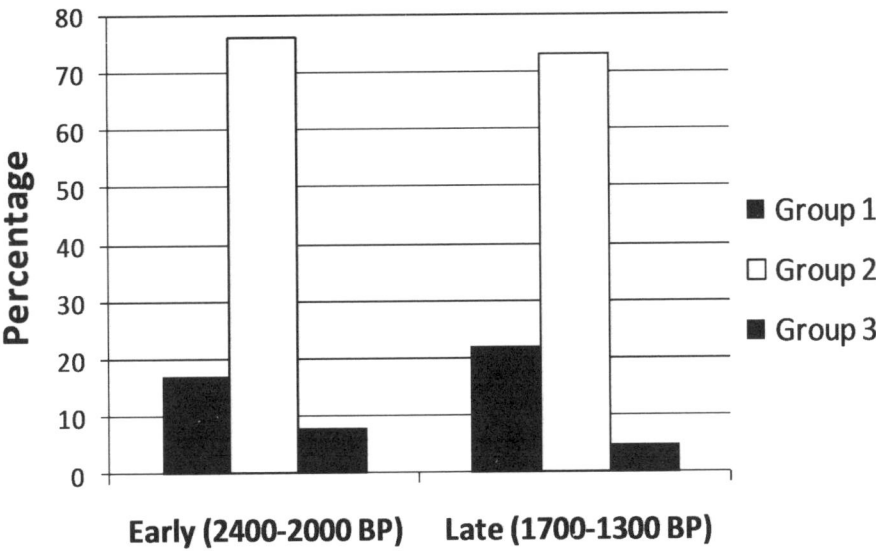

Figure 15.2. Representation of the different ceramic groups in Casa Chávez Montículos during its two phases.

The Ceramic Assemblage from Casa Chávez Montículos

The pottery recovered from the Early and Late phases CChM (Fig. 15.2) is technologically homogeneous, with compact fabrics of irregular colour and both organic and inorganic inclusions (Vidal 2007). However, the different size, form and thickness of the vessels suggest a three-fold division of the material from a function–use perspective. Furthermore, these three groups display some variation in their chronological distribution.

Group 1 is poorly represented in both phases. The ceramics are generally thin walled and incompletely fired with inorganic inclusions and polished surfaces. Some specimens have been found to have external soot deposits with evidence of internal combustion with deposits of animal fat (Vidal 2003). From this, it may be suggested that these vessels functioned primarily as cooking pots, although they could equally have been used for serving, storing or transporting small amounts of foodstuffs or similar materials.

Group 2 is the most plentiful throughout the settlement's occupation, although its representation increases slightly in the later phase of the site. It is difficult to discern a specific function for this group but some functions, such as long-term storage and processing, can be ruled out because of the fragility of walls and the reduced size of the vessels. Some sherds show thin soot deposits that may have resulted from occasional culinary activities. The high representation of this group, together with its form, breakage patterns and generalized disposal would appear to suggest frequent, even daily use, probably related to food consumption practices, as suggested by ethnographic cases (Rice 1987, 293–301).

Group 3, which is characterized by thick walls and simple profiles, seems to be the most appropriate form for long-term storage, as well as the processing of food or other substances. Interestingly, the distribution of this pottery type declines considerably through time. This reduction demands further discussion considering the increased agricultural production of this period – one would expect that this would have also heightened the demands for storage. The possibility that the decline in Group 3 representation can be linked to site-formation processes can be ruled out on the basis of the ceramic's thickness and density, which would have ensured its preservation. Contemporary theft is also improbable due to the low aesthetic appeal of this ceramic group. Instead, the answer to the relative decline in this pottery may be related to the cultural practices defining the vessels' use. The simplest explanation would be that it simply reflects a decline in storage needs; however, the situation may be more complex, given the wider social transformations that were taking place at the time.

The CChM Ceramics in Context

Archaeobotanical studies suggest that through the course of its occupation, CChM witnessed an increase in plant consumption – maize and other vegetables – which was connected to the agricultural intensification of the period (Olivera and Vigliani 1999). A higher reliance on plants may explain why the later levels yielded a larger number of Groups 1 and 2 sherds with soot deposits: maize grains and most dryland vegetables demand long boiling and, consequently, a fire-resistant vessel. However, it might be expected that an increase in vegetable consumption would be accompanied by both an increase in processing tools and storage vessels, but neither is recorded in the later levels at CChM.

Given that evidence for storage containers declines at the time that new sites were being established in the surrounding landscape, we propose that both storage and the initial processing of vegetables, tubers and corns (such as flour) was relocated from residential settlements, like CChM, to cultivation areas (i.e. the nearby site of Bajo del Coypar). Semi-processed food products would then be transported to the tell, according to the needs of the local population. Such a situation would account for the decline in storage containers (Group 3) and the parallel increase in cooking/serving vessels (Groups 1 and 2) seen in the later settlement levels.

Eating, Processing and Storing Food in Arid Andean Highlands

Acknowledgements

To my old ANS research team and The Visual Learning Lab., University of Nottingham. Many thanks to Naomi Sykes for her patience and much-needed suggestions to enhance this paper.

References

Olivera, D. 1997. 'Los primeros pastores de la Puna Sur Argentina: una aproximación a través de su cerámica', *Revista de Arqueología Americana* 13, 69–112. Instituto Panamericano de Geografía e Historia, San José de Costa Rica.
——, Vidal, A. and Grana, L. 2003. 'El sitio Cueva Cacao 1A: hallazgos, espacio y proceso de complejidad en la Puna Meridional (*ca.* 3000 años AP)', *Relaciones de la Sociedad Argentina de Antropología* 28, 257–270.
——, and Vigliani, S. 1999. 'Proceso cultural, uso del espacio y producción agrícola en la Puna Meridional Argentina', *Cuadernos del INAPL* 19, 35–52.
Rice, P. 1987. *Pottery Analysis: A Sourcebook* (Chicago).
Vidal, A. 2003. 'Análisis porosimétrico de materiales cerámicos tempranos del NOA', *Avances en Arqueometría* (Puerto de Santa María), 3–9.
—— 2007. 'Análisis funcional de la cerámica utilitaria en Casa Chávez Montículos (Prov. de Catamarca)', *Shincal* 7, 1–20.

Prehistoric Spoons:
Their Representation in Time and Space

Aixa Vidal, Universidad Complutense de Madrid; Instituto Nacional de Antropología y Pensamiento Latinoamericano
and
M. Soledad Mallía, Universidad de Buenos Aires; INAPL

In modern households, spoons are one of the most common domestic tools, basically used for mixing and consuming liquid foods. Despite, or perhaps because of their familiarity, little thought has been given to the antiquity of these artefact types, and whether their function has remained constant over time. This short paper aims to provide a review of the evidence for spoons in prehistoric Europe, assessing their chronological and spatial distribution, while considering the constraints imposed on their physical or documentary retrieval. By examining their depositional contexts we will offer alternative explanations for the changing roles that spoons may have fulfilled: holding, serving and drinking. Our hope is that this paper might act as a foundation for future functional studies.

Methods

This review is based largely on published works (for references see Vidal and Mallía forthcoming), which present a number of problems in terms of data integrity. In both past and present literature, some artefacts have been identified as 'spoons' because of their morphology. However, other objects of similar shape have been labelled variously as 'ladle' or 'scoop' (see Fig. 16.1). Regardless of their classification, very few analyses have been carried out to determine their actual use and/or contents (Maicas and Vidal 2010; Pascual 1998). To ensure that our study incorporates all possible specimens, we define spoons simply as an artefact with two distinct parts: a bowl deep enough to hold liquids, and a handle of any length and shape. They may be compound tools, such as the presumed spoons made of shell with a wooden handle in the Spanish south-east (Siret 1908), or one-piece artefacts, like the clay spoon found in Cork, Ireland (Grogan and Roche 2007). Such a broad definition widens the number of specimens to be considered, with considerable variety of shapes, raw materials and sizes. It must be assumed that the diversity of spoon types had equally diverse functions – from a large spoon as big as a drinking cup to the tiny cosmetic-holders of ancient Egypt (Baduel 2005) – but we feel that it is necessary to consider the evidence on its broadest scale if we are to understand the finer details of spoon use.

Prehistoric Spoons: Their Representation in Time and Space

Term used/proposed function	Associated residues
'spatula', ' ladle ', 'spurtle'	Ointments
Oil lamps	Lipids
Short-term containers	Pigments (make up), varnish, bitumen/mastic
Cups	Alcoholic beverages?
Measurement units	
Cultic implements	Psychoactives ?

Figure 16.1. Different terms used in the literature for spoon-shaped artefacts and their associated residues.

The compilation presented here is by no means a comprehensive review as some specimens are still to be discovered in established collections, new ones are always being recovered in current excavations and further examples are identified in previously published materials. Some excavation reports are new or ongoing and not yet readily accessible, and older material is sometimes rendered less useful by its lack of either rigorous description or graphic representaton, and by its use of variant terminology. Without illustration, we must rely on the author's identification of the artefact, which may not necessarily match ours. Thus, some so-called spoons in the literature have to be left out of our calculations until new data establishes a qualification for their inclusion.

Chronological Distribution

Archaeological spoons are found in low quantities at various domestic prehistoric sites (Fig. 16.1). The earliest examples date to the Upper Palaeolithic period but specimens are also known from a number of Mesolithic sites (Lillie et al. 2005). Spoons seem to be especially numerous in the Neolithic, when they are made of a range of materials, including clay, shell, bone and wood. However both the frequency of spoons and the range of materials from which they were manufactured appear to decline through the course of the Chalcolithic and Bronze Age (Fig. 16.1).

Geographical Distribution

Figure 16.2 demonstrates that spoons are well represented in the European Mediterranean basin, being particularly abundant in Greece (Björk 1995) and Spain (Pascual 1998), followed by Italy (Fugazzola et al. 2002) and France (Aubin 1989). Furthermore, they were recovered from very diverse settings: drylands and wetlands, fluvial plains and,

Prehistoric Spoons: Their Representation in Time and Space

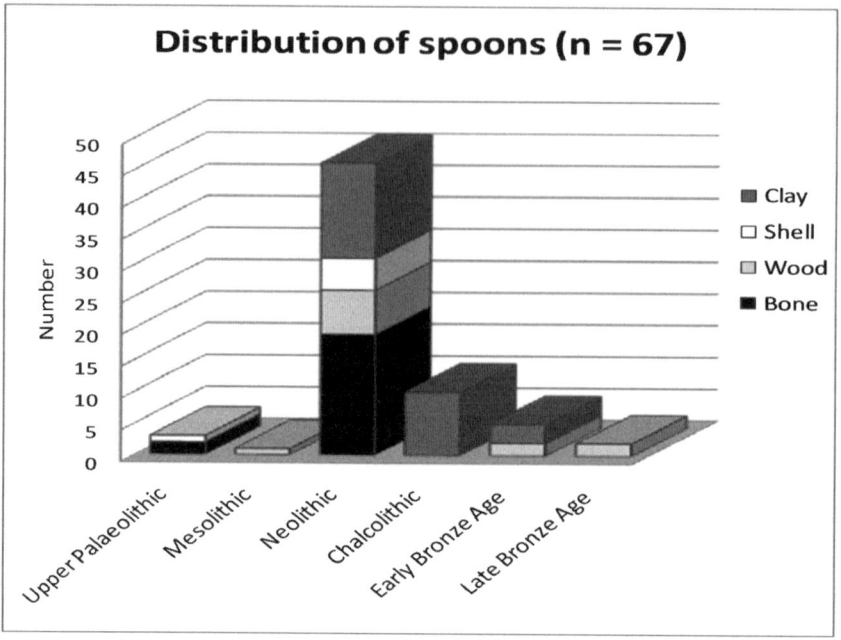

Figure 16.2. The temporal distribution of spoons and their materials of manufacture.

predominantly, caves. Spoons are far less numerous in northern regions although, to some extent, the geographical representation of spoons is influenced by both the materials from which they were manufactured and the conditions in which they were buried.

Northern environments are more favourable to the preservation of wooden materials, with most specimens coming from waterlogged lakesides and bog deposits. However, the frequency of wooden spoons from northern Europe is still low in comparison with the retrieval of wooden vessels in the same area, such as the carved and finely finished legged bowls and dishes. Wooden spoons from northern Europe were made from birch (*Betula* sp.), oak (*Quercus* sp.), alder (*Alnus* sp.), *Prunus* sp., willow (*Salix* sp.) and hazel (*Corylus avellana*), which contrast with the hardwood species – box (*Buxus sempervirens*) and wild olive (*Olea europaea*) – preferred for the manufacture of southern European spoons.

Bone spoons are more durable, which may explain why they are comparatively better represented in earlier periods (Fig. 16.1). They are common finds in eastern Europe, where a number of finely decorated specimens has been recovered. Spoons made from the bones of auroch (*Bos primigenius*) are frequent in Early Neolithic Hungary, and unfinished items were found in Neolithic Poland, while antler spoons are present in Bronze Age Sweden (Czerniak et al. 2003). The outstanding abundance of bone spoons in south-eastern Spain is certainly significant from a regional perspective (Fig. 16.3).

Prehistoric Spoons: Their Representation in Time and Space

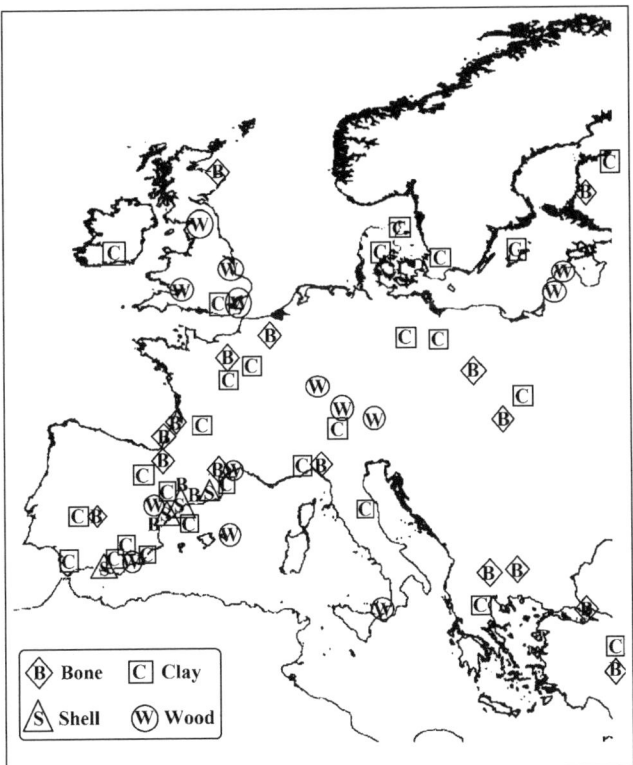

Figure 16.3. The main records of spoons in prehistoric Europe and neighbouring areas, highlighted according to raw material (Vidal & Mallía forthcoming).

The distribution of shell spoons, on the other hand, seems to be biased according to research intensity rather than factors of preservation: spoons have only recently been thoroughly explored, particularly in Spanish contexts. In this region, shell spoons have been found at both inland and coastal sites. Bivalve molluscs such as *Glycymeris* sp., *Cerastoderma* sp. and *Acanthocardia* sp. are frequent raw materials (Maicas and Vidal 2010). Given the morphology and size of the original shell, very little modification was required to convert them into spoons; however, some examples seem to have been substantially altered to improve their suitability as containers rather than being simple utensils or ornaments (Vidal and Maicas, this volume).

Clay spoons have the widest geographical and temporal distribution, being found from the Neolithic to the Bronze Age, from southern Greece to Scandinavia. In the literature these items have sometimes been ambiguously classified as oil lamps, particularly when the absence of the distinctive bowl portion hampers their identification (Fig. 16.1). They are found not only in domestic contexts but also in burials, suggesting they had some significance beyond their role of simple functional tools.

Function and Use

In such a short review it is difficult to consider in any detail the varying uses and significance of this object group but there are some basic patterns that may be discerned. Perhaps the most striking is the comparative abundance of spoons in contexts dating to the Neolithic period. It is tempting to suggest that the Mesolithic/Neolithic transition was characterized not only by the introduction of innovative foods but also by new forms of dining etiquette. It seems feasible that the frequency of spoons reflects a shift from shared to private food consumption, whereby spoons were used either as individual containers or as items to scoop nourishment from larger drink or food vessels, or rather as sizable ladles for individual apportioning in the domestic or workshop sphere. Certainly, the bone spoons from eastern Europe tend to be small in size, suggesting that they may be regarded as individual tools (Gimbutas et al. 1989). However, we should be wary of interpreting these objects with reference to the modern usage of spoons; they may have fulfilled an entirely different role. For instance, in regions where prehistoric spoons are scarce, such as northern Europe, they tend to have been recovered from contexts that seem to be strongly ritual in nature: noteworthy examples include the specimen retrieved from the wetlands of the Sweet Track site in Somerset, England (Coles and Orme 1976) and the example from Mitchelstown, Ireland, associated with a unique anthropomorphic vessel (Grogan and Roche 2007).

Conclusion

The available evidence suggests that the tools we have labelled as 'spoons' were quite frequent in prehistoric times, though the record displays many gaps, especially in some northern areas. Retrieval conditions are partly responsible for the variety of the findings, due to the organic nature of most of the raw materials and the low visibility of some kinds of sites that may have yielded them. Nevertheless, one of the main reasons why spoons are not easily found in the literature is the general lack of publication – or sometimes the low quality of publications issued – by private companies that excavate the sites, and the difficulty of gaining access to institutional materials. Furthermore, in earlier published material, spoons are often classified under unexpected or variant headings, such as spatulae, lamp, small vessel or shovel, making their identification a hard task at best. Despite all these constraints, spoons are worth analysing as they may reveal not only accepted patterns of behaviour but also potential shifts in consumption practices that would enhance our view of social life in the past.

Prehistoric Spoons: Their Representation in Time and Space

Acknowledgements

To Ruth Maicas, Sebastian Guest, The Visual Learning Lab. and Naomi Sykes, University of Nottingham for assistance and funding. Many thanks to an anonymous reviewer for suggestions. This research is part of an independent initiative which aims to document the presence of these artefacts in a wider European context and compile a background database.

References

Aubin, J. 1989. 'Néolithique au quotidien', *Actes XVIº Colloque Interrégional sur le Néolithique. 4 L'alimentation* (Paris), 163–171.

Baduel, N. 2005. 'La question des palettes et du fard', *Dossiers d'Archeologie* 307, 44–51.

Björk, C. 1995. *Early Pottery in Greece. A Technological and Functional Analysis of the Evidence from Neolithic Achilleion Thessaly* (Jonsered).

Coles, A. and Orme, M.1976. 'The Sweet Track Railway site', *Somerset Levels Papers* 2, 34–65.

Czerniak, L., Raczkowski, W. and Sosnowski, W. 2003. 'New prospects for the study of Early Neolithic longhouses in the Polish Lowlands', *Antiquity* 77 (297), Project Gallery http://www.antiquity.ac.uk/projgall/czerniak297/.

Fugazzola, M., Pessina, A. and Tiné V. 2002. *Le Ceramiche Impresse nel Neolitico Antico. Italia e Mediterraneo* (Rome).

Gimbutas, M., Winn, S., Shimbuku, D. 1989. *Achilleion, A Neolithic Settlement in Thessaly, Greece (6400–4600 BC)* (Los Angeles).

Grogan, E. and Roche, H. 2007. *New Routes to the Past: Archaeology and the National Roads Authority Monograph Series* 4 (Dublin).

Lillie, M., Zhilin, M., Shavchenko, S. and Taylor, M. 2005. 'Carpentry dates back to Mesolithic', *Antiquity* 79 (305), Project Gallery http://antiquity.ac.uk/projgall/lillie/index.html.

Maicas, R. and Vidal, A. 2010. 'More than food: beads and shell tools in Late Prehistory in the Spanish Southeast', in *Munibe*, Suplemento 31. Proceedings of the 2nd Archaeomalacology Working Group Meeting (Santander 2008), 168–175.

Pascual, J. 1998. *Utillaje Óseo, Adornos e Idolos Neolíticos Valencianos* (Valencia).

Siret, L. 1908. *Religiones neolíticas de Iberia*. Colección Siret de Arqueología 2 (Almería).

Vidal, A., Mallía, M. forthcoming. 'Good manners at the table: a survey of spoons in Prehistoric Western Europe', *WAC proceedings* (Dublin 2008).